Hypoglycemia in Diabetes

Pathophysiology, Prevalence, and Prevention

3rd Edition

Philip E. Cryer, MD

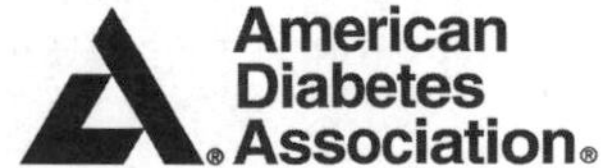

Director, Book Publishing, Abe Ogden; *Managing Editor,* Rebekah Renshaw; *Acquisitions Editor,* Victor Van Beuren; *Production Manager,* Melissa Sprott; *Production Services,* Cenveo Publisher Services; *Cover Design,* Koncept, Inc.; *Printer,* Thomson-Shore.

Printed in the United States of America
1 3 5 7 9 10 8 6 4 2

The suggestions and information contained in this publication are generally consistent with the *Standards of Medical Care in Diabetes* and other policies of the American Diabetes Association, but they do not represent the policy or position of the Association or any of its boards or committees. Reasonable steps have been taken to ensure the accuracy of the information presented. However, the American Diabetes Association cannot ensure the safety or efficacy of any product or service described in this publication. Individuals are advised to consult a physician or other appropriate health care professional before undertaking any diet or exercise program or taking any medication referred to in this publication. Professionals must use and apply their own professional judgment, experience, and training and should not rely solely on the information contained in this publication before prescribing any diet, exercise, or medication. The American Diabetes Association—its officers, directors, employees, volunteers, and members—assumes no responsibility or liability for personal or other injury, loss, or damage that may result from the suggestions or information in this publication.

♾ The paper in this publication meets the requirements of the ANSI Standard Z39.48-1992 (permanence of paper).

Jane Chiang, MD, conducted the internal review of this book to ensure that it meets American Diabetes Association guidelines.

ADA titles may be purchased for business or promotional use or for special sales. To purchase more than 50 copies of this book at a discount, or for custom editions of this book with your logo, contact the American Diabetes Association at the address below or at booksales@diabetes.org.

American Diabetes Association
1701 North Beauregard Street
Alexandria, Virginia 22311

DOI: 10.2337/9781580406499

Library of Congress Cataloging-in-Publication Data

Names: Cryer, Philip E., 1940- , author. | American Diabetes Association, issuing body.
Title: Hypoglycemia in diabetes / Philip E. Cryer.
Description: 3rd edition. | Alexandria : American Diabetes Association, [2016] | Includes bibliographical references and index.
Identifiers: LCCN 2016009040 | ISBN 9781580406499
Subjects: | MESH: Hypoglycemia--physiopathology | Hypoglycemia--epidemiology | Hypoglycemia–prevention & control | Diabetes Complications
Classification: LCC RC662.2 | NLM WK 880 | DDC 616.4/66–dc23
LC record available at http://lccn.loc.gov/2016009040

This book is dedicated to the research nurses, led for a quarter of a century by Carolyn E. Havlin-Cryer, RN, and the following research fellows:

Alan J. Garber, MD, PhD
William L. Clarke, MD
Alan B. Silverberg, MD
Steven A. Leveston, MD
Jack F. Tohmeh, MD
William E. Clutter, MD
Dennis A. Popp, MD
Ann M. Ginsberg, MD, PhD
Pierre Serusclat, MD
Thomas F. Tse, MD
Stephen G. Rosen, MD
Michael A. Berk, MD
Myrlene Staten, MD
David P. Hoelzer, MD
Natalie S. Schwartz, MD
Katherine R. Tuttle, MD
Karen M. Tordjman, MD
Stephen B. Liggett, MD
James C. Marker, PhD
Patrick J. Boyle, MD
Irl B. Hirsch, MD
Simon R. Heller, DM, FRCP
Brian V. Wiethop, MD
Samuel E. Dagogo-Jack, MB/BS, FRCP
Dwight A. Towler, MD, PhD
Chatchalit Rattarasarn, MD
Annemarie Hvidberg, MD, PhD
Tarek Saleh, MD
Carmine G. Fanelli, MD
Deanna Paramore, MD
Fernando Ovalle, MD
Scott A. Segel, MD
Salomon Banarer, MD
Veronica P. McGregor, MD
Michael A. DeRosa, DO
Bharathi Raju, MD
Denise Teves, MD
Ana Maria Arbeláez, MD
Suzanne M. Breckenridge, MD
Benjamin A. Cooperberg, MD
Ranjani P. Ramanathan, MD
Nadia Khoury, MD

These individuals did the bulk of our work.

Contents

Preface to the Third Edition

Diabetes is an increasingly common disease. It is estimated that the prevalence of diabetes will rise from 415 million people in the year 2015 to 642 million people worldwide by the year 2040[1] and that the total diabetes prevalence (diagnosed and undiagnosed cases) will increase from 14% in 2010 to 25–28% of the U.S. population by 2050.[2] The most common forms of the disease are type 1 diabetes (T1D), the result of absolute insulin deficiency from its clinical onset; and type 2 diabetes (T2D), the result of relative insulin deficiency in the setting of insulin resistance early in its course and absolute insulin deficiency later. Approximately 95% of affected people have T2D.

Over time, diabetes can cause unique microvascular complications—retinopathy, nephropathy, and neuropathy—and a substantially increased risk for macrovascular atherosclerotic complications—myocardial infarction, cerebrovascular accidents, and peripheral vascular disease. These long-term complications are undoubtedly multifactorial in origin, but it is now well established, at least for microvascular disease, that hyperglycemia is one important factor. Maintenance of plasma glucose concentrations closer to the nondiabetic range partially prevents or delays microvascular complications in T1D[3,4] and in T2D.[5,6] It may reduce macrovascular complications in T1D[7,8] and T2D,[9] although that remains to be documented.[10]

Unfortunately, with current treatment regimens, it is not possible to maintain euglycemia over a lifetime of diabetes in the vast majority of people with diabetes because of the barrier of iatrogenic (treatment-induced) hypoglycemia.[10–15] Pending the prevention and cure of diabetes, maintenance of euglycemia without hypoglycemia will require new treatment methods that provide plasma glucose regulated insulin replacement or secretion, that is, closed-loop insulin replacement, transplantation of β-cell-containing tissue, or expansion of β-cell mass.

The biochemistry, physiology, and pathophysiology of intermediary metabolism, with a focus on glucoregulation and hypoglycemia, have been reviewed,[11–15,16–18] and the history of hypoglycemia in the 20th century has been summarized.[11] The impact of hypoglycemia was first documented in 1921 when a dog convulsed and then died after injection of extracted insulin; hypoglycemia was recognized to be a complication of insulin treatment of diabetes shortly thereafter.[19]

Hypoglycemia is both a clinical and a physiological term. Unequivocal demonstration of clinical hypoglycemia requires documentation of Whipple's triad[20]: symptoms, signs, or both, consistent with hypoglycemia; a reliably measured low plasma glucose concentration; and resolution of those symptoms and signs after the plasma glucose level is raised.[15] In healthy individuals, symptoms of hypoglycemia develop at an arterialized venous plasma glucose concentration of 50–55 mg/dL (2.8–3.0 mmol/L).[16] From a physiological perspective, however, the glycemic threshold is at a higher glucose level. Arterialized venous plasma glucose concentrations just below the postabsorptive physiological range, that is, <70 mg/dL (<3.9 mmol/L), trigger physiological defenses against falling plasma glucose concentrations, including further decrements in the secretion of insulin and initial increments in the secretion of glucose counterregulatory hormones, such as glucagon and epinephrine.[16] Indeed, the latter higher plasma glucose concentration, with or without symptoms, has been recommended as a pragmatic alert level for people with diabetes who are at high risk for clinical hypoglycemia.[21–24]

This third edition of *Hypoglycemia in Diabetes* is updated and expanded but retains its focus on the clinical problem of hypoglycemia in diabetes. That problem is approached from the perspective of the pathophysiology of glucose counterregulation, the mechanisms that normally effectively prevent or correct hypoglycemia,[16] in T1D and advanced T2D.[12–15,17,18] Insight into that pathophysiology leads to increased understanding of the frequency of, risk factors for, and prevention of iatrogenic hypoglycemia in people with diabetes.

Philip E. Cryer, M.D.
Professor of Medicine Emeritus
Washington University in St. Louis

References

1. International Diabetes Federation. *IDF Diabetes Atlas,* 7th Ed. Brussels, International Diabetes Federation, 2015 (http://www.diabetesatlas.org)
2. Boyle JP, Thompson YJ, Gregg EW, Barker LE, Williamson DF. Projection of the year 2050 burden of diabetes in the U.S. adult population: dynamic modeling of incidence, mortality and prediabetes prevalence. *Popul Health Metr* 2010;8:29–41
3. Diabetes Control and Complications Trial Research Group. The effect of intensive treatment of diabetes on the development and progression of long-term complications in insulin dependent diabetes mellitus. *N Engl J Med* 1993; 329:977–986
4. Diabetes Control and Complications Trial/Epidemiology of Diabetes Interventions and Complications (DCCT/EDIC) Research Group. Retinopathy and nephropathy in patients with type 1 diabetes four years after a trial of intensive therapy. *N Engl J Med* 2000;342:381–389
5. U.K. Prospective Diabetes Study Group (UKPDS). Intensive blood-glucose control with sulphonylureas or insulin compared with conventional treatment and risk of complications in patients with type 2 diabetes (UKPDS 33). *Lancet* 1998; 352:837–853
6. U.K. Prospective Diabetes Study Group (UKPDS). Effect of intensive blood-glucose control with metformin on complications in overweight patients with type 2 diabetes (UKPDS 34). *Lancet* 1998;352:854–865
7. Diabetes Control and Complications Trial/Epidemiology of Diabetes Interventions and Complications (DCCT/EDIC) Research Group. Intensive diabetes treatment and cardiovascular disease in patients with type 1 diabetes. *N Engl J Med* 2005;353:2643–2653
8. Polak JF, Backlund JY, Cleary PA, Harrington AP, O'Leary DH, Lachin JM, Nathan DM for the DCCT/EDIC Research Group. Progression of carotid artery intima-media thickness during 12 years in the Diabetes Control and Complications

Trial/Epidemiology of Diabetes Interventions and Complications (DCCT/EDIC) study. *Diabetes* 2011;60:607–613

9. Holman RR, Paul SK, Bethel MA, Matthews DR, Neil HAW. 10-year follow-up of intensive glucose control with type 2 diabetes. *N Engl J Med* 2008; 359: 1577–1589

10. Cryer PE. Glycemic goals in diabetes: trade-off between glycemic control and iatrogenic hypoglycemia. *Diabetes* 2014;63:2188–2195

11. Cryer PE. *Hypoglycemia: Pathophysiology, Diagnosis and Treatment*. New York, Oxford University Press,1997, p 1–177

12. Cryer PE. Diverse causes of hypoglycemia-associated autonomic failure in diabetes. *N Engl J Med* 2004;350:2272–2279

13. Cryer PE. The barrier of hypoglycemia in diabetes. *Diabetes* 2008;57: 3169–3176

14. Cryer PE. Hypoglycemia in diabetes. In *Textbook of Diabetes,* 4th Edition. Holt RIG, Cockram C, Flyvbjerg A, Goldstein BJ, Eds. Oxford, U.K., Wiley-Blackwell, p. 528–545

15. Cryer PE. Hypoglycemia. In *Williams Textbook of Endocrinology,* 13th Edition. Melmed S, Polonsky KS, Larsen PR, Kronenberg HM, Eds. Philadelphia, Elsevier, 2016, p. 1582–1607

16. Cryer PE. The prevention and correction of hypoglycemia. In *Handbook of Physiology,* Section 7, The Endocrine System. Volume II, The Endocrine Pancreas and Regulation of Metabolism. Jefferson LS, Cherrington AD, Eds. New York, Oxford University Press, p. 1057–1092

17. Cryer PE. Elimination of hypoglycemia from the liver of people with diabetes. *Diabetes* 2011;60:24–27

18. Cryer PE. Mechanisms of hypoglycemia-associated autonomic failure in diabetes. *N Engl J Med* 2013;369:362–372

19. Bliss M. *The Discovery of Insulin*. Chicago, University of Chicago Press, 1984, p. 109, 155, 157–158

20. Whipple AO. The surgical therapy of hyperinsulinism. *J Int Chir* 1938; 3: 237–276

21. American Diabetes Association Workgroup on Hypoglycemia. Defining and reporting hypoglycemia in diabetes. *Diabetes Care* 2005;28:1245–1249

22. Cryer PE. Preventing hypoglycaemia: what is the appropriate glucose alert value? *Diabetologia* 2009;52:35–37

23. Seaquist ER, Anderson J, Childs B, Cryer P, Dagogo-Jack S, Fish L, Heller SR, Rodriguez H, Rosenzweig J, Vigersky R. Hypoglycemia and diabetes: a report of a workgroup of the American Diabetes Association and the Endocrine Society. *Diabetes Care* 2013;36:1384–1395

24. International Hypoglycaemia Study Group. Minimizing hypoglycemia in diabetes. *Diabetes Care* 2015;38:1583–1591

Acknowledgments

The author's original work cited was supported in part by the U.S. Public Health Service, National Institutes of Health grants, including R37 DK27085, MO1 RR00036 (now UL1 RR24992), P60 DK20579, and T32 DK07120, and by research grants and a fellowship award from the American Diabetes Association. The author is grateful for the contributions of his mentors, collaborators, and colleagues; the efforts of the postdoctoral fellows who did the bulk of the work and made the work better by their conceptual input; and the skilled nursing, technical, dietary, and data management and statistical assistance of the staff of the Washington University General Clinical Research Center.

Disclosures

The author has served as a consultant to several pharmaceutical or medical device firms, including Amgen Inc., Bristol-Myers Squibb/AstraZeneca, Calibrium, Johnson & Johnson, Lilly/Boehringer-Ingelheim, MannKind Corp., Marcadia Biotech, Medtronic MiniMed Inc., Merck and Co., Pfizer, Novo Nordisk A/S, Takeda Pharmaceuticals North America, and TolerRx Inc.

1 The Clinical Problem of Hypoglycemia in Diabetes

The Context

Iatrogenic hypoglycemia is the limiting factor in the glycemic management of diabetes.[1–5] First, it causes recurrent morbidity in most people with type 1 diabetes (T1D), and many with advanced (absolute endogenous insulin deficient) type 2 diabetes (T2D), and is sometimes fatal. Second, it compromises physiological and behavioral defenses against subsequent falling plasma glucose concentrations and thus causes a vicious cycle of recurrent hypoglycemia. Third, it generally precludes maintenance of euglycemia over a lifetime of diabetes and thus full realization of the vascular benefits of long-term glycemic control.[6–11] Hypoglycemia is not only common and potentially devastating but also costly.[12]

Because of the barrier of hypoglycemia, no professional treatment guidelines recommend a glycemic goal of euglycemia, that is, a normal hemoglobin A_{1c} (A1C) level, although that undoubtedly would be beneficial with respect to the long-term microvascular complications of diabetes if it could be accomplished safely. For example, the American Diabetes Association[13] recommends an A1C goal of <7% for many nonpregnant adult patients with diabetes, or <7.5% in individuals less than 18 years of age.[14]

Glucose is an obligate metabolic fuel for the brain under physiological conditions.[3–5] Mechanisms have evolved that normally effectively prevent or rapidly correct hypoglycemia despite wide variations in glucose flux into and

DOI: 10.2337/9781580406499.01

out of the circulation (see Chapter 2),[15,16] undoubtedly because of their survival value. Thus, hypoglycemia is a distinctly uncommon clinical event, except in people who use drugs that lower the plasma glucose concentration—specifically, insulin, a sulfonylurea, or a glinide—to treat diabetes.[17]

Clinical hypoglycemia is a plasma glucose concentration low enough to cause symptoms or signs, including impairment of brain function.[17,18] Because the clinical manifestations of hypoglycemia are nonspecific (see Chapter 2), hypoglycemia is documented most convincingly by Whipple's triad [19]: symptoms, signs, or both consistent with hypoglycemia; a low reliably measured plasma glucose concentration; and resolution of the symptoms and signs after the plasma glucose concentration is raised. Because even asymptomatic low plasma glucose concentrations impair defenses against subsequent hypoglycemia (see Chapter 3), hypoglycemia is defined more broadly in people with diabetes: all episodes of abnormally low plasma glucose concentration that expose the individual to potential harm.[20,21] Ideally, people with diabetes should self-monitor their plasma glucose level when they suspect it is low. Because the risk of hypoglycemia is high in patients treated with insulin, a sulfonylurea, or a glinide—and the potential detrimental effects of untreated hypoglycemia outweigh those of unnecessary treatment—a clinical diagnosis of hypoglycemia is reasonable in such patients even in the absence of a glucose measurement, if symptoms develop. Similarly, this diagnosis is reasonable if a low glucose level is monitored, even in the absence of recognized symptoms.

Hypoglycemia in diabetes is generally the result of the interplay of relative or absolute therapeutic (exogenous or endogenous) insulin excess and compromised physiological and behavioral defenses against falling plasma glucose concentrations (see Chapter 3).[1–3,5,22] Thus, it is fundamentally iatrogenic, the result of treatments that raise circulating insulin levels and therefore lower plasma glucose concentrations. Those treatments include insulin or an insulin secretagogue such as a sulfonylurea (glyburide [glibenclamide], glipizide, glimepiride, or gliclazide, among others) or a glinide (nateglinide or repaglinide). Interactions between sulfonylureas and other drugs, including antibiotics, can result in hypoglycemia.[23] Antidiabetic drugs, mostly insulin, were found to be second only to anticoagulants as a cause of emergency hospitalization for adverse drug events in people >65 years of age, and those visits were almost entirely because of hypoglycemia.[24] All people with T1D must be treated with insulin. Many people with T2D ultimately require treatment with insulin.[25] Early in the course of T2D, patients may respond to an insulin secretagogue, with the risk of hypoglycemia. Alternatively, they may respond to drugs that do not raise insulin levels at normal or low plasma glucose concentrations and therefore should not, and probably do not, cause hypoglycemia.[26–28] The latter include the biguanide metformin—which nonetheless has been reported to cause self-reported hypoglycemia[29,30]—thiazolidinediones (e.g., pioglitazone, rosiglitazone), α-glucosidase inhibitors (e.g., acarbose, miglitol), glucagon-like peptide-1 (GLP-1) receptor agonists (e.g., exenatide, liraglutide, albiglutide, lixisenatide, dulaglutide), dipeptidyl peptidase-IV (DPP-IV) inhibitors (e.g., sitagliptin, saxagliptin, vildagliptin, linagliptin, alogliptin), and sodium-glucose cotransporter 2 (SGLT2) inhibitors (e.g., canagliflozin, dapagliflozin, empagliflozin, others). All of these drugs require endogenous insulin secretion to lower plasma glucose concentrations, and insulin secretion declines appropriately as glucose levels fall into the normal range. This decline is true even for the GLP-1 receptor agonists and the DPP-IV inhibitors, which enhance glucose-stimulated insulin secretion (among other actions). They do not stimulate insulin secretion at normal or low plasma glucose levels (i.e., they increase insulin secretion in a glucose-dependent fashion). Indeed, all six categories of drugs—biguanides, thiazolidinediones, α-glucosidase inhibitors, GLP-1 receptor agonists, DPP-IV inhibitors, and SGLT2 inhibitors—would be expected to increase the risk of hypoglycemia if used with an insulin secretagogue or with insulin if the latter drugs suppress mean glycemia. GLP-1 receptor agonists also inhibit glucagon secretion in a glucose-dependent fashion. They decrease it during hyperglycemia and euglycemia but not during hypoglycemia; indeed, they enhance glucagon secretion during hypoglycemia.[31] Even the salicylate salsalate increased the risk of hypoglycemia sixfold when given with a sulfonylurea.[32] The bile acid sequestrant colesevelam and the dopamine receptor agonist bromocriptine should not cause hypoglycemia. Among potential future glucose-lowering drug categories, agents that activate G-protein coupled receptor 40[33] should not cause hypoglycemia, whereas glucokinase activators would cause hypoglycemia.[34,35]

Frequency of Hypoglycemia

If it is shown to accurately and reliably reflect plasma glucose concentrations and is linked to continuous recording of symptoms, continuous subcutaneous glucose monitoring might lead to more detailed knowledge of the precise prevalence and incidence of hypoglycemia in diabetes.[36,37] Pending that, we must rely on estimates (Table 1.1).

Table 1.1—Event Rates for Severe Hypoglycemia (that Requiring the Assistance of Another Person), Expressed as Episodes per 100 Patient-Years, in Insulin-Treated Diabetes

	n	Event rate	Comment
Type 1 Diabetes			
U.K. Hypoglycemia Study Group[38]	57[a] 50[b]	320 110	Prospective multicenter study
MacLeod et al.[39]	544	170	Retrospective clinic survey, randomly selected sample
Donnelly et al.[40]	94	115	Prospective study, population-based random sample
Reichard and Pihl[41]	48	110	Clinical trial, intensive insulin group
DCCT Research Group[6]	711	62	Clinical trial, intensive insulin group
Type 2 Diabetes			
MacLeod et al.[39]	56	73	Retrospective clinic survey, randomly selected sample
U.K. Hypoglycemia Study Group[38]	77[c] 89[d]	70 10	Prospective multicenter study
Akram et al.[42]	401	44	Retrospective clinic survey
Donnelly et al.[40]	173	35	Prospective study, population-based random sample
Henderson et al.[43]	215	28	Retrospective clinic survey, randomly selected sample
Murata et al.[44]	344	21	Prospective study, random Veterans Affairs sample
Saudek et al.[45]	62	18[e]	Clinical trial, multiple insulin injection group
Gürlek et al.[46]	114	15	Retrospective clinic survey
Abraira et al.[47]	75	3	Clinical trial, intensive insulin group
Yki-Järvinen et al.[48]	88	0	Clinical trial, initial insulin therapy
Ohkubo et al.[49]	52	0	Clinical trial, initial insulin therapy

[a]Insulin treatment for >15 years
[b]Insulin treatment for <5 years
[c]Insulin treatment for >5 years
[d]Insulin treatment for <2 years
[e]Definite (8 per 100 patient-years) plus suspected (10 per 100 patient-years) severe hypoglycemia

Studies covering at least 1 year, involving at least 48 patients, and reporting severe hypoglycemia event rates are included. This table was prepared, by the author, for a Clinical Practice Guideline on hypoglycemia in adults (Cryer et al. 2009).

Source: Cryer et al.[17]

Insulin-induced hypoglycemia led to nearly 100,000 emergency department visits annually, and nearly 30,000 hospitalizations annually, in 2007–2011 in the U.S.[50] These data undoubtedly underestimate the iatrogenic hypoglycemia burden because hypoglycemia, even severe temporarily disabling hypoglycemia, most often is cared for outside of emergency departments.

Type 1 Diabetes

Hypoglycemia is a fact of life for most people with T1D (Table 1.1).[1–3,5,6,38–41,51] The average patient suffers untold numbers of asymptomatic episodes, two episodes of symptomatic hypoglycemia per week (thousands of such episodes over a lifetime of diabetes), and one to three episodes of severe, temporarily disabling hypoglycemia, often with seizure or coma, per year.

Given increased recognition of the magnitude of the problem of iatrogenic hypoglycemia in T1D, and practical improvements in the glycemic management of diabetes, over the two decades since the Diabetes Control and Complications Trial (DCCT) was reported in 1993,[6] one might anticipate that hypoglycemia would have become less of a problem. Unfortunately, in contrast to data from observational studies in pediatric T1D,[52,53] no evidence is found in population-based studies. For example, in their study reported in 2007, the U.K. Hypoglycaemia Study Group[38] found the incidence of severe hypoglycemia in patients with T1D treated with insulin for <5 years to be comparable to that in the Stockholm Diabetes Intervention Study[41] (both 110 per 100 patient-years) reported in 1994 and higher than that in the DCCT reported in 1993 (Table 1.1). Remarkably, the U.K. Hypoglycaemia Study Group[38] found the incidence of severe hypoglycemia in patients with T1D treated with insulin for >15 years (320 episodes per 100 patient-years) to be threefold higher than in individuals treated for <5 years (Table 1.1). In addition, an incidence of 300 episodes per 100 patient-years was reported in 2007 in a prospective observational study of 7,067 patients with T1D.[51] Clearly, the frequency of severe hypoglycemia reported from clinical populations is higher than that reported from treatment trials (Table 1.1).[51,54] Notably, a nearly twofold increase in the incidence of symptomatic hypoglycemia with a plasma glucose of <50 mg/dL (2.8 mmol/L) requiring treatment with intravenous glucose was noted in one study from 1997–2000 to 2007–2010 in patients with T1D and T2D.[55]

The distribution of severe hypoglycemia in T1D is skewed. In one series, with an incidence of 130 episodes per 100 patient-years, only 37% of the patients suffered severe hypoglycemia.[56] A reasonable generalization is that 30–40% of patients with T1D suffer one to three episodes of severe hypoglycemia each year.[18]

Hypoglycemia is particularly common during the night.[57,58] Nocturnal plasma glucose concentrations were <63 mg/dL (3.5 mmol/L) in 13 of 29 (45%) prepubertal patients with T1D and the median duration of those low nocturnal glucose concentrations was 4.5 h.[57] In adults treated with contemporary aggressive methods, and with relatively tight glycemic control, one-quarter of all nocturnal plasma glucose concentrations were <70 mg/dL (3.9 mmol/L) and the duration of low values ranged up to 7 h.[58] Six percent of the values were <50 mg/dL (2.8 mmol/L). The extent to which lower rates of nocturnal hypoglycemia detected in T1D by continuous subcutaneous glucose monitoring[59] are a function of the monitoring technique or the patients studied is not known. That technique, however, did not distinguish patients with impaired awareness of hypoglycemia, who had a greater than threefold increased incidence of severe hypoglycemia, from those with normal awareness of hypoglycemia.[60]

Type 2 Diabetes

Overall, hypoglycemia is less frequent in T2D than in T1D (Table 1.1).[38,40,61–63] Hypoglycemia, however, becomes progressively more limiting to glycemic control later in the course of T2D[38,64] Indeed, the frequency of hypoglycemia has been reported to be similar in patients with T2D and patients with T1D matched for duration of insulin therapy.[61] When comparing patients with T2D treated with insulin for <2 years with patients treated with insulin for >5 years, the U.K. Hypoglycaemia Study Group[38] found severe hypoglycemia prevalences of 7 and 25% and incidences of 10 and 70 episodes per 100 patient-years, respectively. The pattern for self-treated hypoglycemia was similar.[38] Thus, although the risk of hypoglycemia is relatively low in the first few years of insulin treatment of T2D (at least with current less than euglycemic glycemic goals), the risk increases substantially, approaching that in T1D, later in the course of T2D.

Because of the difficulty of ascertainment, reported incidences of hypoglycemia in diabetes generally are underestimated. Asymptomatic episodes of hypoglycemia will be missed unless these episodes are detected by routine self–plasma glucose monitoring (or by reliable continuous subcutaneous glucose monitoring). Because the symptoms of hypoglycemia are nonspecific (see Chapter 2), symptomatic episodes may not be recognized as the result of hypoglycemia.[65] Even if they are recognized, mild-to-moderate self-treated episodes are often not long remembered[66–68] and therefore may not be reported accurately at periodic clinic visits. Episodes of severe hypoglycemia (those sufficiently disabling that they require the assistance of another person) are more dramatic events that are much more likely to be recalled[66–68] and therefore reported by the patient or by a close associate. Thus, although they represent only a small fraction of the total hypoglycemic experience, estimates of the incidence of severe hypoglycemia are the most reliable. Arguably, they are also most important, because they pose a high risk for a subsequent serious adverse outcome and dictate consideration of a major change in the therapeutic regimen. In addition, hypoglycemia event rates determined prospectively, particularly if hypoglycemia is the primary outcome in a population-based study, should be more reliable than those determined retrospectively. Although estimates of the incidence of hypoglycemia (Table 1.1) often are derived from clinical treatment trials, there are several limitations to that approach. First, hypoglycemia is not a primary outcome of such trials; therefore, the extent of collection of data concerning hypoglycemia varies. For example, much was learned about the incidence of hypoglycemia in T1D in the DCCT,[69] but the incidence of hypoglycemia in T2D in the U.K. Prospective Diabetes Study (UKPDS) is not known.[30] Second, treatment trials in T2D often are conducted in patients just failing oral hypoglycemic agent therapy and naive to insulin therapy. Such patients are not representative of advanced T2D and are at relatively low risk for hypoglycemia, as mentioned earlier,[38] for pathophysiological reasons developed in Chapter 3. Third, if used exclusively, that approach ignores evidence from clinical experience in diabetes specialist clinics and data from prospective, population-based studies focused on hypoglycemia.

The prospective, population-based study of Donnelly and colleagues[40] indicates that the overall incidence of hypoglycemia in insulin-treated T2D is approximately one-third of that in T1D (Table 1.1). In patients with T1D, the event rates for any hypoglycemia and for severe hypoglycemia were ~4,300 per 100 patient years and 115 per 100 patient-years, respectively. In patients with insulin-treated T2D, the event rates for any hypoglycemia and for severe hypoglycemia were ~1,600 per 100 patient years and 35 per 100 patient-years, respectively. Furthermore, in population-based studies from single hospital regions with known incidences of T1D and T2D, event rates for severe hypoglycemia requiring emergency medical treatment in insulin-treated T2D were ~40%[62] and ~100%[55] of those in T1D. Because the prevalence of T2D is ~20-fold greater than that of T1D, and because many people with T2D ultimately require treatment with insulin,[25] these data suggest that most episodes of iatrogenic hypoglycemia, including severe iatrogenic hypoglycemia, occur in people with T2D. In short, up to 25% of patients with insulin-treated T2D, and <10% of those treated with a sulfonylurea, suffer severe hypoglycemia in a given year.[38,70] Clearly, the magnitude of the problem of hypoglycemia in T2D should not be underestimated.

Compared with that in T1D, the incidence of hypoglycemia is relatively low (at least with currently recommended glycemic goals) during treatment with an insulin secretagogue or even with insulin early in the course of T2D.[38] Hypoglycemia, however, becomes progressively more frequent, with its incidence approaching that in T1D, in patients with longstanding insulin-treated T2D.[38] As developed in Chapter 3, this increase in the frequency of iatrogenic hypoglycemia parallels progressive β-cell failure in T2D and thus development of the pathophysiology of glucose counterregulation—compromised physiological and behavioral defenses against falling plasma glucose concentrations—as patients approach the insulin-deficient end of the spectrum of T2D.[1–3,5,22]

Impact of Hypoglycemia

Iatrogenic hypoglycemia causes recurrent morbidity in most people with T1D and many with advanced T2D and is sometimes fatal.[1–5] Because it generally precludes maintenance of euglycemia over a lifetime of diabetes, and thus full realization of the vascular benefits [6,8–11,71] of glycemic control, the barrier of hypoglycemia may contribute to the most prevalent causes of disabling morbidity and of mortality in diabetes. Finally, hypoglycemia impairs defenses against subsequent hypoglycemia.

Morbidity

Glucose, almost exclusively derived from the circulation, is an obligate metabolic fuel for the brain under physiological conditions (see Chapter 2). Hypoglycemia causes brain fuel deprivation that, if unchecked, results in functional brain failure that typically is corrected after the plasma glucose concentration is raised.[16] Rarely, hypoglycemia results in death.[4]

The physical morbidity of an episode of hypoglycemia ranges from unpleasant symptoms, such as palpitations, tremulousness, anxiety, sweating, hunger, and paresthesias,[72] to cognitive impairments with behavioral changes, seizure, coma, or, rarely, death.[4,16] Physical injuries or transient focal neurological deficits occur rarely. Seemingly complete recovery after an episode of hypoglycemia is the rule. Permanent neurological damage is rare. In monkeys, 5–6 h of blood glucose concentrations <20 mg/dL (1.1 mmol/L) were required for the regular production of clinically overt brain damage.[7.3]

It is conceivable that hypoglycemia, or more likely the responses to hypoglycemia, are a factor in the pathogenesis of macrovascular disease in diabetes. Patients with T1D and recurrent severe hypoglycemia, compared with those without severe hypoglycemia, have been found to have lower flow-mediated brachial artery dilatation and increased carotid and femoral artery intima-media thickness, both markers of preclinical atherosclerosis.[74] Yasunari et al.[75] report that repetitive insulin-induced hypoglycemia accelerated injury-induced neointima formation and cell proliferation in rat carotid artery, an effect attenuated by administration of an α-adrenergic antagonist, indicating that it was mediated by catecholamines released by hypoglycemia. Mechanisms by which responses to hypoglycemia might contribute to macrovascular disease have been summarized in recent studies.[76–78]

Prospective data in youth with T1D indicate that hypoglycemia adversely affects verbal abilities, working memory, and nonverbal processing speed.[79,80] Evidence indicates that subtle but detectable relationships exist between glycemic extremes, including hypoglycemia, and brain function, and structure in youth with T1D.[81] An association between hypoglycemic seizures and a decline in verbal IQ in youth with T1D has been reported.[82] Nonetheless, the results of long-term follow-up of adult DCCT patients[83,84] are to a large extent reassuring. In 1,144 patients with T1D (40% of whom suffered at least one episode of hypoglycemic coma or seizure) followed for a mean of 18 years, hypoglycemia was not associated with a decline in any cognitive domain. Thus, recurrent hypoglycemia does not appear to cause cognitive impairment in young to middle-age adults with T1D.[83,84] Not only did the DCCT/EDIC population not include children, however, but also did not include elderly persons. In the Fremantle study of patients with T2D >70 years of age at baseline, no relationship was found between a history of severe hypoglycemia and cognitive decline during follow-up.[85] However, only 205 patients were followed and only 33 experienced cognitive decline over a mean of 1.6 years. In contrast, a retrospective analysis of data from 16,667 patients with T2D and a mean age of 65 years disclosed a graded relationship between episodes of severe hypoglycemia and dementia risk.[86] The hazard ratios were 1.3, 1.8, and 1.9 for one, two, or three or more episodes of severe hypoglycemia, respectively. Furthermore, a population-based study disclosed an association between a self-reported history of severe hypoglycemia and poorer late-life cognitive ability in people with T2D.[87] Also, 12-year follow-up of older adults with diabetes without dementia at baseline disclosed that those who experienced severe hypoglycemia had a twofold increased risk for dementia and those who developed dementia had a threefold increased risk for subsequent severe hypoglycemia.[88] Additional evidence indicates a bidirectional association between hypoglycemia and dementia in older adults with T2D.[89]

At the very least, an episode of hypoglycemia is a nuisance and a distraction. Hypoglycemia can be embarrassing and can lead to social ostracism or employment discrimination. It can be mistaken for alcohol intoxication or illicit drug use. The resulting aberrant behavior and impaired judgment can lead to offensive acts, and altered psychomotor functions can cause impaired performance of physical tasks (such as driving). Indeed, drivers with both T1D and insulin-treated T2D acknowledge some unsafe driving practices during hypoglycemia.[90] In T1D, hypoglycemia-related driving mishaps have been associated with a history of severe hypoglycemia[91] as well as with a lower A1C level and a history of severe hypoglycemia.[92] The psychological morbidity of iatrogenic hypoglycemia includes fear of an episode (which can be a barrier to glycemic control), guilt about that fear, higher levels of anxiety, and lower levels of overall happiness.[93] Fear of hypoglycemia is common and is associated with the experience of severe hypoglycemia.[18,94]

Mortality

The vast majority of episodes of hypoglycemia, including severe episodes that cause functional brain failure—impaired cognition, aberrant behavior, and even seizure or loss of consciousness—are corrected after the plasma glucose concentration is raised. Prolonged, profound hypoglycemia can cause brain death, but that is rare and most fatal episodes are the result of other mechanisms, presumably largely cardiac arrhythmias.[4,16,77,95,96]

Despite some exceptions,[97,98] evidence is abundant that iatrogenic hypoglycemia, caused by treatment of diabetes with insulin or a sulfonylurea, is associated with death, and substantive evidence indicates that iatrogenic hypoglycemia is one cause of death of people with diabetes.[4,99,100] Obviously, hypoglycemia is not the cause of death that occurs in the absence of hypoglycemia. Furthermore, because there are many other causes of hypoglycemia including critical illnesses,[5,17] all hypoglycemia is not iatrogenic hypoglycemia. Finally, an association between the occurrence of hypoglycemia and death in a population does not establish that hypoglycemia was the cause of all, or even any, of the deaths.

The Toronto investigators' insulin extract sometimes killed diabetic dogs, and they found that convulsions and deaths following insulin extract administration could be prevented by intravenous glucose administration in rabbits early in 1922.[101] Deaths of patients from what were identified as "insulin reactions" were reported in 1923.[101] In addition, there is a high death rate in experimental insulin-induced hypoglycemia.[102–104] Thus, there is no doubt that iatrogenic hypoglycemia can kill.

There is substantial epidemiological evidence of associations between iatrogenic hypoglycemia and mortality, or potentially mortal events, in diabetes. That includes greater mortality in patients treated with sulfonylureas compared with metformin[105–108] and associations between hypoglycemia and acute cardiovascular events,[109,110] including ventricular tachycardia[111] and increased mortality in insulin-treated patients.[112–114] Meta-analyses not only have documented associations between hypoglycemia and cardiovascular mortality but also, based on bias analyses, have suggested that the associations were not the result of confounding comorbidities—that is, that hypoglycemia was likely causal of cardiovascular mortality.[115,116] Additional reports have noted an association between severe iatrogenic mortality and death in insulin-treated diabetes.[117–119] Reports of associations between severe hypoglycemia and adverse molecular events have been discussed.[120]

Severe hypoglycemia was associated with increased mortality in seven randomized controlled trials of intensive glycemic therapy, two in intensive care unit (ICU) patients,[121,122] four in patients with T2D,[123–126] and one in patients with T1D.[119] These epidemiological associations do not establish a casual connection. Nonetheless, the consistent pattern in all seven trials increases the probability that hypoglycemia was the cause of some of the deaths. Furthermore, although increased mortality in the intensive glycemic therapy limb of

ACCORD might have been the result of some unidentified nonglycemic aspect of the intensive glycemic therapy regimens,[123] the intensive glycemic therapy regimen was the same in both limbs in the ICU patients.[121] Only the glycemic goals differed.

Although older series indicated that 2 to 4% of patients with T1D died forom hypoglycemia,[127–129] more recent series indicate hypoglycemic mortality rates of 4%,[130] 7%,[131] 8%,[119] and 10%.[132] Indeed, hypoglycemia at the time of death of a patient with T1D has been documented by continuous glucose monitoring (Figure 1.1).[133]

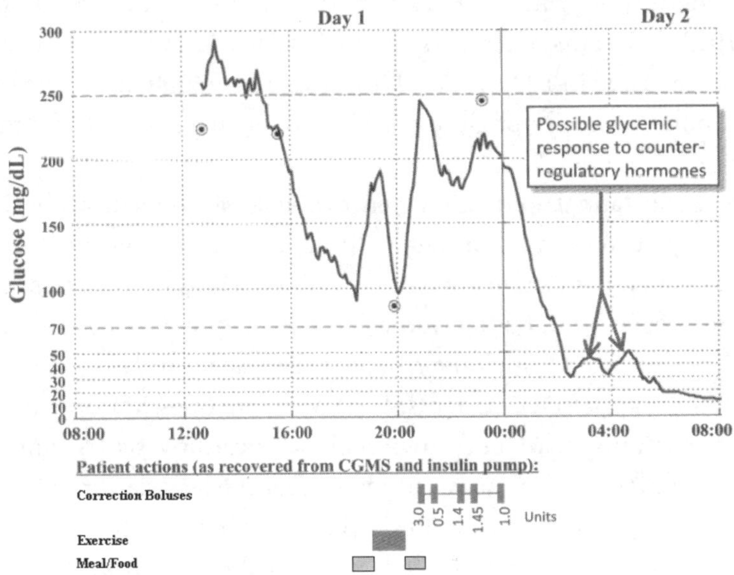

Figure 1.1—Continuous subcutaneous glucose monitoring data from a patient with type1 diabetes the afternoon, evening, and night before he was found dead in bed. The self plasma glucose monitoring values obtained by the patient are shown by the four circles. The times of insulin boluses, exercise, and food ingestion are also shown.

Source: From Tanenberg et al.[133] with permission from the American Association of Clinical Endocrinologists.

Interestingly, McCoy and colleagues[134] reported a 3.4-fold higher mortality, without a difference in the Charlson comorbidity index, in patients with T1D or T2D who self-reported severe hypoglycemia (that requiring the assistance of another person) 5 years earlier. Clearly, whatever the absolute rate, there is an iatrogenic mortality rate in T1D.

There is also an iatrogenic mortality rate in T2D.[62,135,136] Of the evaluable deaths in the ACCORD trial, four (1%) were judged definitely or probably due to hypoglycemia and an additional 38 (9%) were judged possibly due to hypoglycemia.[136] Finally, an association between low (as well as high) A1C levels and mortality in people with diabetes has been documented in several reports.[137–146]

The clinical implication of these data is that overly aggressive glucose-lowering therapy may cause excess mortality in diabetes—that is, there is a limit to the degree of glycemic control that can be maintained safely with currently available methods.[4] One might ask: What is an acceptable iatrogenic hypoglycemic mortality rate in diabetes, particularly in view of the decreasing incidences of diabetes-related complications, including acute myocardial infarction and stroke, in recent decades?[147] The possible mechanisms of lethal hypoglycemia-induced ventricular arrhythmias[4,77,95,96,148–151] are discussed in Chapter 3. The relevance of these findings to glycemic goals and the extent to which technological advances might permit lower glycemic goals in the future are discussed in Chapter 6.

Summary

Hypoglycemia is a problem for many people with diabetes that has not been solved. It is fundamentally iatrogenic, the result of therapeutic hyperinsulinemia. Because of the effectiveness of normal defenses against falling plasma glucose concentrations (see Chapter 2), hypoglycemia is relatively uncommon early in the course of T2D (and is uncommon very early—the "honeymoon" period—in T1D). Hypoglycemia becomes more common over time as those defenses become compromised (see Chapter 3). Understanding the latter pathophysiology leads to insight into the risk factors for (see Chapter 4), definition and classification of (see Chapter 5), and prevention or treatment of (see Chapter 6) iatrogenic hypoglycemia in diabetes.

References

1. Cryer PE. Diverse causes of hypoglycemia-associated autonomic failure in diabetes. *N Engl J Med* 2004;350:2272–2279
2. Cryer PE. The barrier of hypoglycemia in diabetes. *Diabetes* 2008;57:3169–3176
3. Cryer PE. Hypoglycemia in diabetes. In *Textbook of Diabetes.* 4th ed. Holt RIG, Cockram C, Flyvbjerg A, Goldstein BJ, Eds. Oxford, U.K., Wiley-Blackwell, 2010, p. 528–545
4. Cryer PE. Glycemic goals in diabetes: trade-off between glycemic control and iatrogenic hypoglycemia. *Diabetes* 2014;63:2188–2195
5. Cryer PE. Hypoglycemia. In *Williams Textbook of Endocrinology.* 13th ed. Melmed S, Polonsky KS, Larsen PR, Kronenberg HM, Eds. Philadelphia, Elsevier, 2016, p.1582–1607.
6. Diabetes Control and Complications Trial Research Group (DCCT). The effect of intensive treatment of diabetes on the development and progression of long-term complications in insulin dependent diabetes mellitus. *N Engl J Med* 1993;329:977–986
7. Diabetes Control and Complications Trial/Epidemiology of Diabetes Interventions and Complications (DCCT/EDIC) Research Group. Retinopathy and nephropathy in patients with type 1 diabetes four years after a trial of intensive therapy. *N Engl J Med* 2000;342:381–389
8. Diabetes Control and Complications Trial/Epidemiology of Diabetes Interventions and Complications (DCCT/EDIC) Research Group. Intensive diabetes treatment and cardiovascular disease in patients with type 1 diabetes. *N Engl J Med* 2005;353:2643–2653
9. U.K. Prospective Diabetes Study Group (UKPDS). Intensive blood-glucose control with sulphonylureas or insulin compared with conventional treatment and risk of complications in patients with type 2 diabetes (UKPDS 33). *Lancet* 1998;352:837–853
10. U.K. Prospective Diabetes Study Group (UKPDS). Effect of intensive blood-glucose control with metformin on complications in overweight patients with type 2 diabetes (UKPDS 34). *Lancet* 1998;352:854–865
11. Holman RR, Paul SK, Ethel MA, Matthews DR, Neil HAW. 10-year follow-up of intensive glucose control in type 2 diabetes. *N Engl J Med* 2008;359: 1577–1589

12. Quilliam BJ, Simeone JC, Ozbay AB, Kogut SJ. The incidence and costs of hypoglycemia in type 2 diabetes. *Am J Manag Care* 2011;17:673–680

13. American Diabetes Association. Standards of medical care in diabetes–2015. *Diabetes Care* 2015;38(Suppl. 1):S1–S93

14. Chiang JL, Kirkman MS, Laffel LMB, and Peters AL, on behalf of the Type 1 Diabetes Sourcebook Authors. Type 1 diabetes through the life span: a position statement of the American Diabetes Association. *Diabetes Care* 2014;37: 2034–2054

15. Cryer PE. The prevention and correction of hypoglycemia. In *Handbook of Physiology.* Section 7, The Endocrine System. Vol. II, The Endocrine Pancreas and Regulation of Metabolism. Jefferson LS, Cherrington AD, Eds. New York, Oxford University Press, 2001, p. 1057–1092

16. Cryer PE. Hypoglycemia, functional brain failure, and brain death. *J Clin Invest* 2007;117:868–870

17. Cryer PE, Axelrod L, Grossman AB, Heller SR, Montori VM, Seaquist ER, Service FJ. Evaluation and management of adult hypoglycemic disorders. *J Clin Endocrinol Metab* 2009;94:709–728

18. International Hypoglycaemia Study Group. Minimizing hypoglycemia in diabetes. *Diabetes Care* 2015;38:1583–1591

19. Whipple AO. The surgical therapy of hyperinsulinism. *J Int Chir* 1938;3: 237–276

20. American Diabetes Association Workgroup on Hypoglycemia. Defining and reporting hypoglycemia in diabetes. *Diabetes Care* 2005;28:1245–1249

21. Seaquist ER, Anderson J, Childs B, Cryer P, Dagogo-Jack S, Fish L, Heller SR, Rodriguez H, Rosenzweig J, Vigersky R. Hypoglycemia and diabetes: a report of a workgroup of the American Diabetes Association and the Endocrine Society. *Diabetes Care* 2013;36:1384–1395

22. Cryer PE. Mechanisms of hypoglycemia-associated autonomic failure in diabetes. *N Engl J Med* 2013;369:362–372

23. Parekh TM, Raji M, Lin YL, Tan A, Kuo YF, Goodwin JS. Hypoglycemia after antimicrobial drug prescription for older patients using sulfonlyureas. *JAMA Intern Med* 2014;174:1605–1612

24. Budnitz DS, Lovegrove MC, Shehab N, Richards CL. Emergency hospitalizations for adverse drug events in older Americans. *N Engl J Med* 2011;365:2002–2012

25. Turner RC, Cull CA, Frighi V, Holman RR, UK Prospective Diabetes Study (UKPDS) Group. Glycemic control with diet, sulfonylurea, metformin, or insulin in patients with type 2 diabetes mellitus: progressive requirement for multiple therapies (UKPDS 49). *JAMA* 1999;281:2005–2012

26. Ferrannini E, Ramos SJ, Salsali A, Tang W, List JF. Dapagliflozin monotherapy in type 2 diabetic patients with inadequate glycemic control by diet and exercise. A randomized, double-blind, placebo-controlled, phase 3 trial. *Diabetes Care* 2010;33:2217–2224

27. Tschope D, Bramlage P, Binz C, Krekler M, Plate T, Deeg E, Gitt AK. Antidiabetic pharmacotherapy and anamnestic hypoglycemia in a large cohort of type 2 diabetic patients an analysis of the DiaRegis registry. *Cardiovasc Diabetol* 2011;10:66

28. Mearns ES, Sobieraj DM, White CM, Saulsberry WJ, Kohn CG, Doleh Y, Zaccaro E, Coleman CI. Comparative efficacy and safety of antidiabetic drug regimens added to metformin monotherapy in patients with type 2 diabetes: a network meta-analysis. *PLoS One* 2015;10:e0125879

29. U.K. Prospective Diabetes Study Group (UKPDS). Overview of 6 years of therapy of type II diabetes: a progressive disease.*Diabetes* 1995;44:1249–1258

30. Wright AD, Cull CA, MacLeod KM, Holman RR, for the UKPDS Group. Hypoglycemia in type 2 diabetic patients randomized to and maintained on monotherapy with diet, sulfonylurea, metformin, or insulin for 6 years from diagnosis: UKPDS 73. *J Diabetes Complications* 2006;20:395–401

31. Dunning BS, Foley JS, Ahrén B. Alpha cell function in health and disease: influence of glucagon-like peptide-1. *Diabetologia* 2005;48:1700–1713

32. Goldfine AB, Fonseca V, Jablonski KA, Chen YD, Tipton L, Staten MA, Shoelson SE, for the Targeting Inflammation Using Salsalate in Type 2 Diabetes Study Team-2013. Salicylate (salsalate) in patients with type 2 diabetes: a randomized trial. *Ann Intern Med* 2013;159:1–12

33. Burant CF, Viswanathan P, Marcinak J, Cao C, Vakilynejad M, Xie B, Leifke E. TAK-875 versus placebo or glimepiride in type 2 diabetes mellitus: a phase 2, randomized, double-blind, placebo-controlled trial. *Lancet* 2012;379: 1403–1411

34. Meininger GE, Scott R, Alba M, Shentu Y, Luo E, Amin H, Davies MJ, Kaufman KD, Goldstein BJ. Effects of MK-0941, a novel glucokinase activator, on glycemic control in insulin-treated patients with type 2 diabetes. *Diabetes Care* 2011;34: 2560–2566

35. Matschinsky FM, Zelent B, Doliba N, Li C, Vanderkooi JM, Naji A, Sarabu R, Grimsby J. Glucokinase activators for diabetes therapy. *Diabetes Care* 2011; 34(Suppl. 2):S236–S243

36. Juvenile Diabetes Research Foundation (JDRF) Continuous Glucose Monitoring Study Group. Continuous glucose monitoring and intensive treatment of type 1 diabetes. *N Engl J Med* 2008;359:1464–1476

37. Cooke D, Hurel SJ, Casbard A, Steed L, Walker S, Meredith S, Nunn AJ, Manca A, Sculpher M, Barnard M, Kerr D, Weaver JU, Ahlquist J, Newman SP. Randomized controlled trial to assess the impact of continuous glucose monitoring on HbA_{1c} in insulin-treated diabetes (MITRE Study). *Diabet Med* 2009;26:540–547

38. U.K. Hypoglycaemia Study Group (UK Hypo Group). Risk of hypoglycaemia in types 1 and 2 diabetes: effects of treatment modalities and their duration. *Diabetologia* 2007;50:1140–1147

39. MacLeod KM, Hepburn DA, Frier BM. Frequency and morbidity of severe hypoglycaemia in insulin-treated diabetic patients. *Diabet Med* 1993;10:238–245

40. Donnelly LA, Morris AD, Frier BM, Ellis JD, Donnan PT, Durrant R, Band MM, Reekie G, Leese GP, for the DARTS/MEMO Collaboration. Frequency and predictors of hypoglycaemia in type 1 and insulin-treated type 2 diabetes: a population-based study. *Diabet Med* 2005;22:749–755

41. Reichard P, Pihl M. Mortality and treatment side-effects during long-term intensified conventional insulin treatment in the Stockholm Diabetes Intervention Study. *Diabetes* 1994;43:313–317

42. Akram K, Pedersen-Bjergaard U, Carstensen B, Borch-Johnsen K, Thorsteinsson B. Frequency and risk factors for severe hypoglycaemia in insulin-treated type 2 diabetes: a cross sectional survey. *Diabet Med* 2006;23:750–756

43. Henderson JN, Allen KV, Deary IJ, Frier BM. Hypoglycaemia in insulin-treated type 2 diabetes: frequency, symptoms and impaired awareness. *Diabet Med* 2003; 20:1016–1021

44. Murata GH, Duckworth WC, Shah JH, Wendel CS, Mohler MJ, Hoffman RM. Hypoglycemia in stable, insulin-treated veterans with type 2 diabetes: a prospective study of 1662 episodes. *J Diabetes Complications* 2005;19:10–17

45. Saudek CD, Duckworth WC, Giobbie-Hurder A, Henderson WG, Henry RR, Kelley DE, Edelman SV, Zieve FJ, Adler RA, Anderson JW, Anderson RJ, Hamilton BP, Donner TW, Kirkman MS, Morgan NA. Implantable insulin

pump vs. multiple dose insulin for non-insulin dependent diabetes mellitus: a randomized clinical trial. *JAMA* 1996;276:1322–1327

46. Gürlek A, Erbas T, Gedik O. Frequency of severe hypoglycemia in type 1 and type 2 diabetes during conventional insulin therapy. *Exp Clin Endocrinol Diabetes* 1999;107:220–224

47. Abraira C, Colwell JA, Nuttall FQ, Swain CT, Nagel NJ, Comstock JP, Emanuele NV, Levin SR, Henderson W, Lee HS. Veterans Affairs Cooperative Study on Glycemic Control and Complications in Type II Diabetes (VA CSCM). *Diabetes Care* 1995;18:1113–1123

48. Yki-Järvinen H, Ryysy L, Nikkilä K, Tulokas T, Vanamo R, Heikkilä M. Comparison of bedtime insulin regimens in patients with type 2 diabetes mellitus. *Ann Intern Med* 1999;130:389–396

49. Ohkubo Y, Kishikawa H, Araki E, Miyata T, Isami S, Motoyoshi S, Kojima Y, Furuyoshi N, Shichiri M. Intensive insulin therapy prevents the progression of diabetic microvascular complications in Japanese patients with non-insulin dependent diabetes mellitus: a randomized prospective 6-year study. *Diabetes Res Clin Pract* 1995;28:103–117

50. Geller AI, Shehab N, Lovegrove MC, Kegler SR, Weidenbach KN, Ryan GJ, Budnitz DS. National estimates of insulin-related hypoglycemia and errors leading to emergency department visits and hospitalizations. *JAMA Intern Med* 2014;174:678–686

51. Lüddeke H-J, Sreenan S, Aczel S, Maxeiner S, Yeniqun M, Kozlovski P, Gydesen H, Dornhorst A, on behalf of the PREDICTIVE Study Group. PREDICTIVE—A global, prospective observational study to evaluate insulin detemir treatment in types 1 and 2 diabetes: baseline characteristics and predictors of hypoglycemia from the European cohort. *Diabetes Obes Metab* 2007;9:428–434

52. Cooper MN, O'Connell SM, Davis EA, Jones TW. A population-based study of risk factors for severe hypoglycaemia in a contemporary cohort of childhood-onset type 1 diabetes. *Diabetologia* 2013;56:2164–2170

53. Fredheim S, Johansen A, Thorsen SU, Kremke B, Nielsen LB, Olsen BS, Lyngsøe L, Sildorf SM, Pipper S, Mortensen HB, Johannesen J, Svensson J, the Danish Society for Diabetes in Childhood and Adolescence. Nationwide reduction in the frequency of severe hypoglycemia by half. *Acta Diabetol* 2014;52:591–599

54. Weinstock RS, Xing D, Maahs DM, Michels A, Rickels MR, Peters AL, Bergenstal RM, Harris B, Dubose SN, Miller KM, Beck RW, Network TDEC. Severe

hypoglycemia and diabetic ketoacidosis in adults with type 1 diabetes: results from the T1D Exchange clinic registry. *J Clin Endocrinol Metab* 2013;98:3411–3419

55. Holstein A, Patzer OM, Machalke K, Holstein JD, Stumvoll M, Kovacs P. Substantial increase in incidence of severe hypoglycemia between 1997–2000 and 2007–2010. *Diabetes Care* 2012;35:972–975

56. Pedersen-Bjergaard U, Pramming S, Heller SR, Wallace TM, Rasmussen AK, Jorgensen HV, Matthews DR, Hougaard P, Thorsteinsson B. Severe hypoglycaemia in 1076 adult patients with type 1 diabetes: influence of risk markers and selection. *Diabetes Metab Res Rev* 2004;20:479–486

57. Matyka KA, Wigg L, Pramming S, Stores G, Dunger DB. Cognitive function and mood after profound nocturnal hypoglycaemia in prepubertal children with conventional insulin treatment for diabetes. *Arch Dis Child* 1999;81:138–142

58. Raju B, Arbeláez AM, Breckenridge SM, Cryer PE. Nocturnal hypoglycemia in type 1 diabetes: an assessment of preventive bedtime treatments. *J Clin Endocrinol Metab* 2006;91:2087–2092

59. Juvenile Diabetes Research Foundation (JDRF) Continuous Glucose Monitoring Study Group.—Prolonged nocturnal hypoglycemia is common during 12 months of continuous glucose monitoring in children and adults with type 1 diabetes. *Diabetes Care* 2010;33:1004–1008

60. Choudhary P, Geddes J, Freeman JV, Emery CJ, Heller SR, Frier BM. Frequency of biochemical hypoglycaemia in adults with type 1 diabetes with and without impaired awareness of hypoglycaemia: no identifiable difference using continuous glucose monitoring. *Diabet Med* 2010;27:666–672

61. Hepburn DA, MacLeod KM, Pell AC, Scougal IJ, Frier BM. Frequency and symptoms of hypoglycaemia experienced by patients with type 2 diabetes treated with insulin. *Diabet Med* 1993;10:231–237

62. Holstein A, Egberts EH. Risk of hypoglycaemia with oral antidiabetic agents in patients with type 2 diabetes. *Exp Clin Endocrinol Metab* 2003;111:405–414

63. Leese GP, Wang J, Broomhall J, Kelly P, Marsden A, Morrison W, Frier BM, Morris AD, DARTS/MEMO Collaboration. Frequency of severe hypoglycemia requiring emergency treatment in type 1 and type 2 diabetes: a population based study of health service resource use. *Diabetes Care* 2003;26:1176–1180

64. U.K. Prospective Diabetes Study Group (UKPDS). United Kingdom Prospective Diabetes Study 24: a six year, randomized, controlled trial comparing sulfonylurea,

insulin and metformin therapy in patients with newly diagnosed type 2 diabetes that could not be controlled with diet therapy. *Ann Intern Med* 1998;128:165–175

65. Clarke WL, Cox DJ, Gonder-Frederick LA, Julian D, Schlundt D, Polonsky W. Reduced awareness of hypoglycemia in IDDM adults: a prospective study of hypoglycemia frequency and associated symptoms. *Diabetes Care* 1995;18:517–522

66. Pramming S, Thorsteinsson B, Bendtson I, Binder C. Symptomatic hypoglycaemia in 411 type 1 diabetic patients. *Diabet Med* 1991;8:217–222

67. Pedersen-Bjergaard U, Pramming S, Thorsteinsson B. Recall of severe hypoglycemia and self-estimated state of awareness in type 1 diabetes. *Diabetes Metab Res Rev* 2003;19:232–240

68. Akram K, Pedersen-Bjergaard U, Carstensen B, Borch-Johnsen K, Thorsteinsson B. Prospective and retrospective recording of severe hypoglycaemia, and assessment of hypoglycaemia awareness in insulin-treated type 2 diabetes. *Diabet Med* 2009;26:1306–1308

69. Diabetes Control and Complications Trial Research Group (DCCT). Hypoglycemia in the Diabetes Control and Complications Trial. *Diabetes* 1997;46:271–286

70. Edridge CL, Dunkley AJ, Bodicoat DH, Rose TC, Gray LJ, Davies MJ, Kunti K. Prevalence and incidence of hypoglycaemia in 532,542 people with type 2 diabetes on oral therapies and insulin: a systematic review and meta-analysis of population based studies. *PLoS ONE* 2015;10:e0126427

71. The Diabetes Control and Complications Trial/Epidemiology of Diabetes Interventions and Complications Research Group. Retinopathy and nephropathy in patients with type 1 diabetes four years after a trial of intensive therapy. *N Engl J Med* 2000;342:381–389

72. Towler DA, Havlin CE, Craft S, Cryer PE. Mechanism of awareness of hypoglycemia: perception of neurogenic (predominantly cholinergic) rather than neuroglycopenic symptoms. *Diabetes* 1993;42:1791–1798

73. Kahn KJ, Myers RE. Insulin induced hypoglycaemia in the non-human primate. I. Clinical consequences. In *Brain Hypoxia*. Brierley JB, Meldrum BS, Eds. London, William Heinemann Medical Books, 1971, p. 185–194

74. Giménez M, Gilabert R, Monteagudo J, Alonso A, Casamitjana R, Paré C, Conget I. Repeated episodes of hypoglycemia as a potential aggravating factor for preclinical atherosclerosis in subjects with type 1 diabetes. *Diabetes Care* 2011;34: 198–203

75. Yasunari E, Mita T, Opsonic Y, Azuma K, Goto H, Ohmura C, Kanazawa A, Kawamori R, Fujitani Y, Watada H. Repetitive hypoglycemia increases circulating adrenaline level with resultant worsening of intimal thickening after vascular injury in male goto-kakizaki rat carotid artery. *Endocrinology* 2014;155:2244–2253

76. Younk LM, Davis SN. Hypoglycemia and vascular disease. *Clin Chem* 2011;57: 258–260

77. Frier BM, Schernthaner G, Heller SR. Hypoglycemia and cardiovascular risks. *Diabetes Care* 2011;34(Suppl. 2):S132–S137

78. Chow E, Heller SR. Pathophysiology of the effects of hypoglycemia on the cardiovascular system. *Diabetic Hypogly* 2012;5:3–8

79. Lin A, Northam EA, Rankins D, Werther GA, Cameron FJ. Neuropsychological profiles of young people with type 1 diabetes 12 yr after disease onset. *Pediatr Diabetes* 2010;11:235–243

80. Blasetti A, Chiuri RM, Tocco AM, Di Giulio C, Mattei PA, Ballone E, Chiarelli F, Verrotti A. The effect of recurrent severe hypoglycemia on cognitive performance in children with type 1 diabetes: a meta-analysis. *J Child Neurol* 2011;26:1383–1391

81. Arbeláez AM, Semenkovich K, Hershey T. Glycemic extremes in youth with T1DM: the structural and functional integrity of the developing brain. *Pediatr Diabetes* 2013;14:541–553

82. Lin A, Northam EA, Werther GA, Cameron FJ. Risk factors for decline in IQ in youth with type 1 diabetes over 12 years from diagnosis/ illness onset. *Diabetes Care* 2015;38:236–242

83. Jacobson AM, Musen G, Ryan CM, Silvers N, Cleary P, Waberski B, Burwood A, Weinger K, Bayless M, Dahms W, Harth J, for the Diabetes Control and Complications Trial, Epidemiology of Diabetes Intervention and Complications Study Research Group. Long-term effect of diabetes and its treatment on cognitive function. *N Engl J Med* 2007;356:1842–1852

84. Jacobson AM, Ryan CM, Cleary PA, Waberski BH, Weinger K, Musen G, Dahms W, DCCT/EDIC Research Group. Biomedical risk factors for decreased cognitive functioning in type 1 diabetes: an 18 year follow-up of the Diabetes Control and Complication Trial (DCCT) cohort. *Diabetologia* 2011;54:245–255

85. Bruce DG, Davis WA, Casey GP, Clarnette RM, Brown SGA, Jacobs IG, Almeida OP, Davis TME. Severe hypoglycaemia and cognitive impairment in older patients with diabetes: the Fremantle Diabetes Study. *Diabetologia* 2009;52:1808–1815

86. Whitmer RA, Karter AJ, Yaffe K, Quesenberry CP Jr, Selby JV. Hypoglycemic episodes and risk of dementia in older patients with type 2 diabetes mellitus. *JAMA* 2009;301:1565–1572

87. Aung PP, Strachan MWJ, Frier BM, Butcher I, Deary IJ, Price JF on behalf of the Edinburgh Type 2 Diabetes Study Investigators. Severe hypoglycaemia and late-life cognitive ability in older people with type 2 diabetes: the Edinburgh Type 2 Diabetes Study. *Diabet Med* 2012;29:328–336

88. Yaffe K, Falvey CM, Hamilton N, Harris TB, Simonsick EM, Strotmeyer ES, Shorr RI, Metti A, Schwartz AV, Health ABCS. Association between hypoglycemia and dementia in a biracial cohort of older adults with diabetes mellitus. *JAMA Intern Med* 2013;173:1300–1306

89. Feinkohl I, Aung PP, Keller M, Robertson CM, Morling JR, McLachlan S, Deary IJ, Frier BM, Strachan MW, Price JF, on behalf of the Edinburgh Type 2 Diabetes Study (ET2DS) Investigators. Severe hypoglycemia and cognitive decline in older people with type 2 diabetes: the Edinburgh Type 2 Diabetes study. *Diabetes Care* 2014;37:507–515

90. Bell D, Huddart A, Krebs J. Driving and insulin-treated diabetes: comparing practices in Scotland and New Zealand. *Diabet Med* 2010;27:1093–1095

91. Cox DJ, Fort D, Gonder-Frederick L, Clarke W, Mazze R, Weinger K, Ritterband L. Driving mishaps among individuals with type 1 diabetes. A prospective study. *Diabetes Care* 2009;32:2177–2180

92. Redelmeier DA, Kenshole AB, Ray JG. Motor vehicle crashes in diabetic patients with tight glycemic control: a population-based case control analysis. *PLoS Med* 2009;6:e1000192

93. Jacobson AM. The psychological care of patients with insulin-dependent diabetes mellitus. *N Engl J Med* 1996;344:1249–1253

94. Beléndez M, Hernández-Mijares A. Beliefs about insulin as a predictor of fear of hypoglycaemia. *Chronic Illn* 2009;5:250–256

95. Cryer PE. Hypoglycemia-Associated autonomic failure in diabetes: maladaptive, adaptive, or both? *Diabetes* 2015;64:2322–2323

96. Chow E, Bernjak A, Williams S, Fawdry RA, Hibbert S, Freeman J, Sheridan PJ, Heller SR. Risk of cardiac arrhythmias during hypoglycemia in patients with type 2 diabetes and cardiovascular risk. *Diabetes* 2014;63:1738–1747

97. Kosiborod M, Inzucchi SE, Goyal A, Krumholz HM, Masoudi FA, Xiao L, Spertus JA. Relationship between spontaneous and iatrogenic hypoglycemia and

mortality in patients hospitalized with acute myocardial infarction. *JAMA* 2009;301:1556–1564

98. Boucai L, Southern WN, Zonszein J. Hypoglycemia-associated mortality is not drug-associated but linked to comorbidities. *Am J Med* 2011;124:1028–1035

99. Cryer PE. Death during intensive glycemic therapy of diabetes: mechanisms and implications. *Am J Med* 2011;124:993–996

100. Cryer PE. Severe hypoglycemia predicts mortality in diabetes. *Diabetes Care* 2012;35:1814–1816

101. Bliss M. *The Discovery of Insulin.* Chicago, University of Chicago Press, 1984, p. 109, 155, 157–158

102. Auer RN. Progress review: hypoglycemic brain damage. *Stroke* 1986;17:699–708

103. Suh SW, Hamby AM, Swanson RA. Hypoglycemia, brain energetic and hypoglycemic neuronal death. *GLIA* 2007;55:1280–1286

104. Reno CM, Daphna-Iken D, Chen YS, VanderWeele J, Jethi K, Fisher SJ. Severe hypoglycemia-induced lethal cardiac arrhythmias are mediated by sympathoadrenal activation. *Diabetes* 2013;62:3570–3581

105. Schramm TK, Gislason GH, Vaag A, Rasmussen JN, Folke F, Hansen ML, Fosbøl EL, Køber L, Norgaard ML, Madsen M, Hansen PR, Torp-Pedersen C. Mortality and cardiovascular risk associated with different insulin secretagogues compared with metformin in type 2 diabetes, with or without a previous myocardial infarction: a nationwide study. *Eur Heart J* 2011;32:1900–1908

106. Pantalone KM, Kattan MW, Yu C, Wells BJ, Arrigain S, Jain A, Atreja A, Zimmerman RS. Increase in overall mortality risk in patients with type 2 diabetes receiving glipizide, glyburide or glimepiride monotherapy versus metformin: a retrospective analysis. *Diabetes Obes Metab* 2012;14:803–809

107. Li Y, Hu Y, Ley SH, Rajpathak S, Hu FB. Sulfonylurea use and incident cardiovascular disease among patients with type 2 diabetes: prospective cohort among women. *Diabetes Care* 2014;37:3106–3113

108. Monami M, Genovese S, Manucci E. Cardiovascular safety of sulfonylureas: a meta-analysis of randomized clinical trials. *Diabetes Obes Metab* 2013;15: 938–953

109. Goldman D. The electrocardiogram in insulin shock. *Arch Int Med* 1940;66: 93–108

110. Johnston SS, Conner C, Aagren M, Smith DM, Bouchard J, Brett J. Evidence linking hypoglycemic events to an increased risk of acute cardiovascular events in patients with type 2 diabetes. *Diabetes Care* 2011;34:1164–1170

111. Chelliah YR. Ventricular arrhythmias associated with hypoglycaemia. *Anaesth Intensive Care* 2000;28:698–700

112. Hsu PF, Sung SH, Cheng HM, Yeh JS, Liu WL, Chan WL, Chen CH, Chou P, Chuang SY. Association of clinical symptomatic hypoglycemia with cardiovascular events and total mortality in type 2 diabetes: a nationwide population-based study. *Diabetes Care* 2013;36:894–900

113. Garg R, Hurwitz S, Turchin A, Trivedi A. Hypoglycemia, with or without insulin therapy, is associated with increased mortality among hospitalized patients. *Diabetes Care* 2013;36:1107–1110

114. Khunti K, Davies M, Majeed A, Thorsted BL, Wolden ML, Paul SK. Hypoglycemia and risk of cardiovascular disease in insulin-treated people with type 1 diabetes and type 2 diabetes: a cohort study. *Diabetes Care* 2015;38:316–322

115. Goto A, Arah OA, Goto M, Terauchi Y, Noda M. Severe hypoglycaemia and cardiovascular disease: systematic review and meta-analysis with bias analysis. *BMJ* 2013;347:f4533

116. Yeh JS, Sung S-H, Huang HM, Yang H-L, You L-K, Chuang S-Y, Huang P-C, Hsu P-F, Cheng H-M, Chen C-H. Hypoglycemia and risk of vascular events and mortality: a systematic review and meta-analysis. *Acta Diabetol* 2015. doi:10.1007/s00592-95-0803-3

117. Heller SR, Amiel SA, Khunti K, International Hypoglycemia Study Group. Hypoglycemia, a global cause for concern. *Diabetes Res Clin Pract* 2015;110:229–232

118. Cooper MN, de Klerk NH, Jones TW, Davis EA. Clinical and demographic risk factors associated with mortality during early adulthood in a population-based cohort of childhood-onset type 1 diabetes. *Diabet Med* 2014;31:1550–1558

119. Diabetes Control and Complications Trial/Epidemiology of Diabetes Interventions and Complications (DCCT/EDIC) Research Group. Association between 7 years of intensive treatment of type 1 diabetes and long-term mortality. *JAMA* 2015;313:45–53

120. Bedenis R, Price AH, Robertson CM, Morling JR, Frier BM, Strachan MWJ, Price JF. Association between severe hypoglycemia, adverse macrovascular

events, and inflammation in the Edinburgh type 2 diabetes study. Diabetes Care 2014;37:3301–3308

121. Finfer S, Liu B, Chittock DR, Norton R, Myburgh JA, McArthur C, Mitchell I, Foster D, Dhingra V, Henderson WR, Ronco JJ, Bellomo R, Cook D, McDonald E, Dodek P, Hebert PC, Heyland DK, Robinson BG. Hypoglycemia and risk of death in critically ill patients. *N Engl J Med* 2012;367:1108–1118

122. Macrae D, Grieve R, Allen E, Sadique Z, Morris K, Pappachan J, Parslow R, Tasker RC, Elbourne D, for the CHiP Investigators. A randomized trial of hyperglycemic control in pediatric intensive care. *N Engl J Med* 2014;370:107–118

123. Action to Control Cardiovascular Risk in Diabetes Study Group (ACCORD). Effects of intensive glucose lowering in type 2 diabetes. *N Engl J Med* 2008;358:2545–2559

124. ADVANCE Collaborative Group (ADVANCE). Intensive blood glucose control and vascular outcomes in patients with type 2 diabetes. *N Engl J Med* 2008;358:2560–2572

125. Duckworth W, Abraira C, Moritz T, Reda D, Emanuele N, Reaven PD, et al. for the Veterans Affairs Diabetes Therapy (VADT) Investigators. Glucose control and vascular complications in veterans with type 2 diabetes. *N Engl J Med* 2009;360:129–139

126. ORIGIN Trial Investigators. Does hypoglycemia increase the risk of cardiovascular events? A report from the ORIGIN trial. *Eur Heart J* 2013;34:3137–3144

127. Deckert T, Poulsen JE, Larsen M. Prognosis of diabetics with diabetes before the age of 31. I. Survival, cause of deaths and complications. *Diabetologia* 1978;14:363–370

128. Tunbridge WMG. Factors contributing to deaths of diabetics under 50 years of age. *Lancet* 1981;2:569–572

129. Laing SP, Swerdlow AJ, Slater SD, Botha JL, Burden AC, Waugh NR, Smith AWM, Hill RD, Bingley PJ, Patterson CC, Qiao Z, Keen H. The British Diabetic Association Cohort Study. I. All-cause mortality in patients with insulin-treated diabetes mellitus. *Diabet Med* 1999;16:459–465

130. Patterson CC, Dahlquist G, Harjutsalo V, Joner G, Feltbower RG, Svensson J, Schober E, Gyürüs E, Castell C, Urbonaité B, Rosenbauer J, Iotova V, Thorsson AV, Soltész G. Early mortality in EURODIAB population-based cohorts of type 1 diabetes diagnosed in childhood since 1989. *Diabetologia* 2007;50:2439–2442

131. Feltbower RG, Bodansky HJ, Patterson CC, Parslow RC, Stephenson CR, Reynolds C, McKinney PA. Acute complications and drug misuse are important causes of death for children and young adults with type 1 diabetes. *Diabetes Care* 2008;31:922–926

132. Skrivarhaug T, Bangstad H-J, Stene LC, Sandvik L, Hanssen KF, Joner G. Long-term mortality in a nationwide cohort of childhood-onset type 1 diabetic patients in Norway. *Diabetologia* 2006;49:298–305

133. Tanenberg RJ, Newton CA, Drake AJ III. Confirmation of hypoglycemia in the "dead-in-bed" syndrome, as captured by a retrospective continuous glucose monitoring system. *Endocr Pract* 2010;16:244–248

134. McCoy R, Shah ND, Van Houton HK, Wermers RA, Smith SA. Increased mortality of patients with diabetes reporting severe hypoglycemia. *Diabetes Care* 2012;35:1897–1901

135. Gerich JE. Oral hypoglycemic agents. *N Engl J Med* 1989;321:1231–1245

136. Bonds DE, Miller ME, Bergenstal RM, Buse JB, Byington RP, Cutler JA, Dudl RJ, Ismail-Beigi F, Kimel AR, Hoogwerf B, Horowitz KR, Savage PJ, Seaquist ER, Simmons DL, Sivitz WI, Speril-Hillen JM, Sweeney ME. The association between symptomatic, severe hypoglycaemia and mortality in type 2 diabetes: retrospective epidemiological analysis of the ACCORD study. *BMJ* 2010;340:b4909

137. Currie CJ, Peters JR, Tynan A, Evans M, Heine RJ, Bracco OL, Zagar T, Poole CD. Survival as a function of HbA_{1c} in people with type 2 diabetes: a retrospective cohort study. *Lancet* 2010;375:481–489

138. Colayco DC, Niu F, McCombs JS, Cheetham TC. A1C and cardiovascular outcomes in type 2 diabetes. A nested case-control study. *Diabetes Care* 2011;34:77–83

139. Huang ES, Liu JY, Moffet HN, John PM, Karter AJ. Glycemic control, complications, and death in older diabetic patients. *Diabetes Care* 2011;34:1329–1336

140. Shurraw S, Hemmelgarn B, Lin M, Majumdar SR, Klarenbach S, Manns B, Bello A, James M, Turin TC, Tonelli T, for the Alberta Kidney Disease Network. Association between glycemic control and adverse outcomes in people with diabetes mellitus and chronic kidney disease. *Arch Intern Med* 2011;171:1920–1927

141. Ricks J, Molnar MZ, Kovesdy CP, Shah A, Nissenson AR, Williams M, Kalantar-Zadeh K. Glycemic control and cardiovascular mortality in hemodialysis patients with diabetes. *Diabetes* 2012;61:708–715

142. Skriver MV, Stovring H, Kristensen JK, Charles M, Sandbaek A. Short-term impact of HbA_{1c} on morbidity and all-cause mortality in people with type 2 diabetes: a Danish population-based observational study. *Diabetologia* 2012;55:2361–2370

143. Ramirez SP, McCullough KP, Thumma JR, Nelson RG, Morgenstern H, Gillespie BW, Inaba M, Jacobson SH, Vanholder R, Pisoni RL, Port FK, Robinson BM. Hemoglobin A_{1c} levels and mortality in the diabetic hemodialysis population: findings from the Dialysis Outcomes and Practice Patterns Study (DOPPS). *Diabetes Care* 2012;35:2527–2532

144. Weinstock RS, Xing D, Maahs DM, Michels A, Rickels MR, Peters AL, Bergenstal RM, Harris B, Dubose SN, Miller KM, Beck RW, Network TDEC. Severe hypoglycemia and diabetic ketoacidosis in adults with type 1 diabetes: results from the T1D Exchange clinic registry. *J Clin Endocrinol Metab* 2013;98:3411–3419

145. Schoenaker DA, Simon D, Chaturvedi N, Fuller JH, Soedamah-Muthu SS, Group EPCS. Glycemic control and all-cause mortality risk in type 1 diabetes patients: The EURODIAB Prospective Complications Study. *J Clin Endocrinol Metab* 2014;99:800–807

146. Karges B, Rosenbauer J, Kapellen T, Wagner VM, Schober E, Karges W, Holl RW. Hemoglobin A1c levels and risk of severe hypoglycemia in children and young adults with type 1 diabetes from Germany and Austria: a trend analysis in a cohort of 37,539 patients between 1995 and 2012. *PLoS Medicine* 2014;11: e1001742

147. Gregg EW, Li Y, Wang J, Burrows NR, Ali MK, Rolka D, Williams DE, Geiss L. Changes in diabetes-related complications in the United States, 1990–2010. *N Engl J Med* 2014;370:1514–1523

148. Lee SP, Yeoh L, Harris ND, Davies CM, Robinson RT, Leathard A, Newman C, Macdonald IA, Heller SR. Influence of autonomic neuropathy on QTc interval lengthening during hypoglycemia in type 1 diabetes. *Diabetes* 2004;53:1535–1542

149. Adler GK, Bonyhay I, Failing H, Waring E, Dotson S, Freeman R. Antecedent hypoglycemia impairs cardiovascular function. Implications for rigorous glycemic control. *Diabetes* 2009;58:360–366

150. Laitinen T, Lyyra-Laitinen T, Huopio H, Vauhkonen I, Halonen T, Hartikainen J, Niskanen L, Laakso M. Electrocardiographic alterations during hyperinsulinemic hypoglycemia in healthy subjects. *Ann Noninvasive Electrocardiol* 2008;13:97–105

151. Nordin C. The case for hypoglycaemia as a proarrhythmic event: basic and clinical evidence. *Diabetologia* 2010;53:1552–1561

2 The Physiology of Glucose Counterregulation

Hypoglycemia and the Brain

Glucose is an obligate oxidative fuel for the brain under physiological conditions.[1–6] Although the adult human brain constitutes only ~2% of body weight, it accounts for ~20% of whole-body glucose utilization. Thus, survival of the brain, and therefore the individual, requires a virtually continuous supply of glucose to the brain.

Neurons normally oxidize lactate as well as glucose, but that is largely lactate derived from glucose within the brain; it is mostly glucose transported from the circulation into the brain but is partly that derived from glycogen in astrocytes.[7–9] The brain can use fuels other than glucose from the circulation if their circulating levels rise high enough to enter the brain in quantity. A commonly cited example is ketone bodies that are elevated during prolonged fasting[10] and during breast-feeding in infants.[11] Another example is lactate that is sufficiently elevated during vigorous exercise.[12] Nonetheless, among the potential substrates that normally circulate, including β-hydroxybutyrate and lactate, only injection of glucose has been found to rescue the brain of a hypoglycemic animal.[1,13]

At elevated, physiological, or slightly subphysiological (e.g., 65 mg/dL [3.6 mmol/L]) plasma glucose concentrations, the rate of blood-to-brain

DOI: 10.2337/9781580406499.02

glucose transport exceeds the rate of brain glucose metabolism.[14,15] Indeed, plasma glucose concentrations <54 mg/dL (3.0 mmol/L) appear to be required to decrease the cerebral metabolic rate of glucose.[16–18] Thus, all of the glucose required to provide oxidative fuel to the brain can be accounted for by glucose from the circulation.[19,20] The balance of the glucose transported into the brain is either stored as (astrocytic) glycogen or transported back into the circulation.

Direct studies of human brain substrate utilization during hypoglycemia are limited. In a study of rather brief (<40 min) but substantial (43 mg/dL [2.4 mmol/L]) hypoglycemia in healthy humans, brain glucose uptake accounted for ~90% of brain oxygen consumption, and there was no net uptake of lactate or pyruvate, β-hydroxybutyrate, or any of nine amino acids.[19] In another study of more sustained (<120 min) and nearly as substantial (54 mg/dL [3.0 mmol/L]) hypoglycemia in healthy humans, brain lactate uptake increased slightly, but accounted for no more than 25% of the calculated brain energy deficit.[20] There was no net uptake of alanine or leucine. Thus, among the potential alternative fuels that circulate, some evidence suggests that the brain switches from net release to net uptake of lactate during hypoglycemia. Brain lactate uptake is directly related to the plasma lactate concentration[21] and blood-to-brain lactate transport increases when plasma lactate levels are raised to high concentrations by vigorous exercise[12] or by lactate infusion coupled with exercise.[22] It is thought that such lactate oxidation might support 5–10% of neuronal metabolic needs.[23]

Interestingly, in a study employing ^{13}C magnetic resonance spectroscopy during [^{13}C]glucose infusion in eight healthy humans, van de Ven et al.[17] found the incorporation of glucose metabolites within the brain to be similar during euglycemia and hypoglycemia (54 mg/dL [3.0 mmol/L]); calculated tricarboxylic acid cycle rates were 0.48±0.03 and 0.43±0.08 $\mu mol \cdot g^{-1} \cdot min.^{-1}$, respectively. The failure to find a significant decrease in brain oxidative metabolism during hypoglycemia might have been the result of *1*) a small sample size, *2*) measurement in only one region of the brain (the occipital cortex), or *3*) increased oxidation of an alternative fuel such as lactate,[23] although van de Ven et al.[16] considered the latter unlikely. Alternatively, it could be that the glycemic threshold for a decrease in brain oxidative metabolism (as opposed to that for a decrease in blood-to-brain glucose transport) is lower than the plasma glucose level of 54 mg/dL (3.0 mmol/L) studied. The latter interpretation has been supported. The findings, in humans, that *1*) at a plasma glucose concentration of 54 mg/dL (3.0 mmol/L) brain oxidative metabolism is not reduced;[16] 2) the relationship between plasma and brain glucose concentrations during euglycemia and hypoglycemia is linear and its extrapolation suggests that the brain glucose concentration would become zero (when brain glucose metabolism would have to cease) only at a plasma glucose concentration of about ≤36 mg/dL (2.0 mmol/L);[17] and 3) the cerebral metabolic rate of glucose, measured with [1-^{11}C]glucose positron emission tomography, is reduced only at a plasma glucose concentration of 45 mg/dL (2.5 mmol/L)[18] indicate that the glycemic threshold for a decrease in brain glucose metabolism is <54 mg/dL (3.0 mmol/L) but >45 mg/dL (2.5 mmol/L).

At some level of hypoglycemia—when the rate of blood-to-brain glucose transport becomes limiting to that of brain glucose metabolism—astrocytic glycogen could be a reserve source of glucose that fuels astrocytes and (largely as lactate produced by glycolysis of glycogen-derived glucose) neurons.[24] That reserve is limited, however. The brain glycogen concentration is ~1% of that in liver and 10% of that in skeletal muscle. On the basis of rates of brain glucose metabolism measured with [1-^{11}C]glucose and positron emission tomography in healthy humans of 0.17 μmol•g^{-1}•min^{-1}[14,15] and a brain glycogen content measured with [1-^{13}C]glucose and magnetic resonance spectroscopy in healthy humans of 3.5 μmol/g glucosyl units,[24] one can calculate that glycogen in the adult human brain could support brain oxidative metabolism for ~20 min if brain glycogen were to become the sole source of glucose (and thus lactate). (That 20-min oxidative reserve from glycogen calculated from human data is remarkably similar to the finding of compound action potential failure of mouse optic nerves 15.9±0.4 min after initial exposure to glucose-free artificial cerebrospinal fluid.[25]) Even if blood-to-brain glucose transport were to account for 90% of brain glucose metabolism during mild-to-moderate hypoglycemia,[14,15,19,20] the 10% supply of brain glycogen-derived glucose (and lactate) would be exhausted in ~200 min.

Because the brain cannot synthesize glucose, use physiological levels of circulating nonglucose fuels effectively, or store more than a 20-min supply as glycogen, the brain requires a virtually continuous supply of glucose from the circulation. Because facilitated blood-to-brain glucose transport (mediated by GLUT-1) is a direct function of the arterial plasma glucose concentration, maintenance of the plasma glucose concentration at or above the normal range is required. At low plasma glucose concentrations, functional brain failure (and, if hypoglycemia is profound and prolonged, brain death) occurs.[2]

Responses to Hypoglycemia

Falling plasma glucose concentrations elicit a characteristic sequence of responses in humans.[26–28] These are shown diagrammatically in Figure 2.1 and are detailed in Table 2.1. The earliest physiological response is a decrease in insulin secretion. That decrease occurs as plasma glucose levels decline within the physiological range. The secretion of glucose counterregulatory (plasma glucose–raising) hormones, including glucagon and epinephrine, increases as plasma glucose concentrations fall just below the postabsorptive physiological range. Lower glucose levels cause symptoms. Even lower levels cause functional brain failure.[2] Prolonged, very low levels can cause brain death.[2,29]

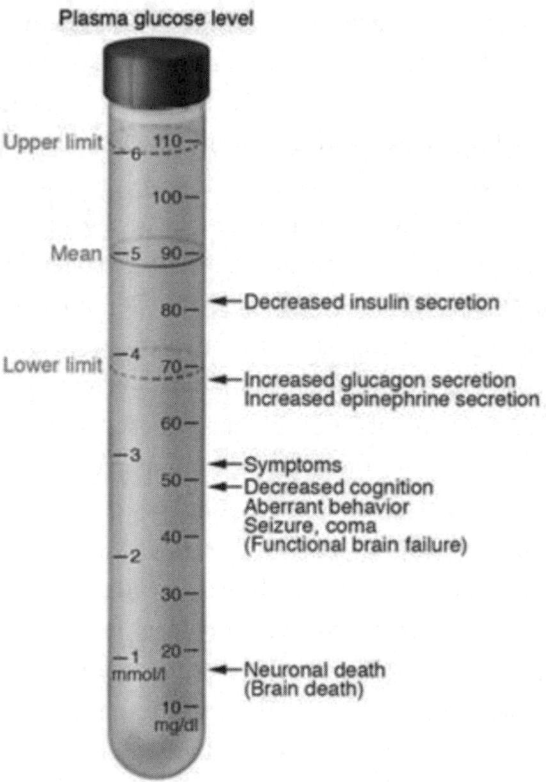

Figure 2.1—Sequence of responses to falling plasma glucose concentrations in humans.

Source: From Cryer[2] with permission from the American Society for Clinical Investigation.

Table 2.1—Physiological Responses to Decreasing Plasma Glucose

Response	Glycemic threshold* [mg/dl(mmol/l)]	Physiological effects	Role in prevention or correction of hypoglycemia (glucose counterregulation)
↓ Insulin	80–85 (4.4–4.7)	↑R_a (↓R_d)	Primary glucose regulatory factor, first defense against hypoglycemia
↑ Glucagon	65–70 (3.6–3.9)	↑R_a	Primary glucose counterrgulatory factor, second defense against hypoglycemia
↑ Epinephrine	65–70 (3.6–3.9)	↑R_a, ↓R_c	Involved, critical when glucagon is deficient, third defense aganist hypoglycemia
↑ Cortisol and growth hormone	65–70 (3.6–3.9)	↑R_a, ↓R_c	Involved, not critical
Symptoms	50–55 (2.8–3.1)	↑Exogenous glucose	Prompt behavioral defense (food ingestion)
↓ Cognition	<50 (<2.8)	—	Compromises behavioral defense

*Arterialized venous, not venous, plasma glucose concentrations. R_a rate of glucose appearance, glucose production by the liver and kidneys; R_d rate of glucose disappearance, glucose utilization by insulin-sensitive tissues such as muscle (no direct effect on central nervous system glucose utilization); R_c rate of glucose clearance by insulin-sensitive tissues.

The evidence that the glycemic threshold for a decrease in brain glucose metabolism is normally <54 mg/dL (3.0 mmol/L),[16–18] discussed earlier, indicates that initialization of the neuroendocrine responses to hypoglycemia is a signaling event and not the result of a decrease in brain glucose metabolism.

Clinical Manifestations of Hypoglycemia

Symptoms and signs of hypoglycemia are not specific.[30] Thus, hypoglycemia is documented most convincingly by Whipple's triad[31]: symptoms, signs, or both consistent with hypoglycemia; a low reliably measured plasma glucose concentration; and resolution of those symptoms and signs after the plasma glucose level is raised.[32] A requirement for formal documentation of Whipple's triad—including a laboratory measurement of a low plasma glucose concentration—is important for the initial demonstration that a hypoglycemic disorder exists in patients without diabetes, because such disorders are rare.[6,32] On the other hand, in patients with diabetes treated with insulin, a sulfonylurea, or a glinide, the likelihood that a given symptomatic episode is the result of hypoglycemia is high (see Chapter 1). Ideally, such patients should estimate their plasma glucose concentrations with a monitor when they suspect their glucose level is low. In reality, sometimes this monitoring is not practical and often it is not done. Nonetheless, it could be reasoned that the detrimental effects of brief erroneous treatment for suspected hypoglycemia are less than those of failure to treat an episode of bona fide hypoglycemia.[2]

Symptoms

Symptoms of hypoglycemia are categorized as neuroglycopenic—those that are the direct result of brain glucose deprivation per se—and neurogenic (or autonomic)—those that are largely the result of the perception of physiological changes caused by the central nervous system (CNS)–mediated sympathoadrenal discharge triggered by hypoglycemia(Figure 2.1 and Table 2.1).[2–4,6,26–28,30,33,34] There is a semantic issue here. Neurogenic symptoms are initiated by glucose deprivation at peripheral and central sensors (i.e., by neuroglycopenia). Their generation, however, includes activation of sympathoadrenal outflow from the brain through the spinal cord to preganglionic neurons innervating the adrenal medullae and sympathetic postganglionic neurons, and they are largely sympathetic neural in origin.[34] Neuroglycopenic manifestations of hypoglycemia include cognitive impairments, behavioral changes, and psychomotor abnormalities, and, at lower plasma glucose levels, seizure and coma—all examples of functional brain failure.[2] Ultimately, after profound, prolonged hypoglycemia, they include brain death.[2]

Neurogenic manifestations of hypoglycemia include both adrenergic and cholinergic symptoms.[30] These are largely the result of sympathetic neural rather than adrenomedullary activation, because bilaterally adrenalectomized individuals experience typical neurogenic symptoms.[34] Adrenergic symptoms—mediated largely by norepinephrine released from sympathetic postganglionic neurons but perhaps also to some extent by circulating epinephrine released from the adrenal medullae—include palpitations, tremor, and anxiety or arousal.[30,34] Cholinergic symptoms—mediated largely by acetylcholine released from sympathetic postganglionic neurons—include sweating, hunger, and paresthesias.[30,34] This classification is based on the effects of adrenergic and cholinergic antagonists.[30] To the extent that those antagonists enter the brain, some of these symptoms (e.g., anxiety or arousal and hunger[35]) may be mediated through central as well as peripheral mechanisms. Nonetheless, electroencephalographic changes and cognitive dysfunction during hypoglycemia higher brain functions are no different in patients with diabetes and clinical hypoglycemia unawareness (see Chapter 3), who have attenuated sympathoadrenal and symptomatic responses to hypoglycemia, and in patients with intact awareness of hypoglycemia.[36] Principal components analysis leads to a somewhat different classification of the symptoms of hypoglycemia.[33,37]

Awareness of hypoglycemia is largely the result of the perception of neurogenic symptoms. It is reduced substantially by combined adrenergic and cholinergic antagonism in humans.[30] Thus, it follows that hypoglycemia unawareness in people with diabetes (see Chapter 3) is largely the result of reduced sympathetic neural, rather than adrenomedullary, activation during hypoglycemia. It is true that patients endorse both neurogenic and neuroglycopenic symptoms of hypoglycemia,[38] but the extent to which they interpret neuroglycopenic symptoms as indicative of hypoglycemia is unclear.

Signs

Pallor and diaphoresis (caused by adrenergic cutaneous vasoconstriction and cholinergic stimulation of sweat glands, respectively) are common signs of hypoglycemia. Heart rate and systolic blood pressure are raised, but usually not greatly. Neuroglycopenic manifestations are often observable. Transient neurological deficits sometimes occur.

Systemic Glucose Balance

Normally, rates of glucose flux into and out of the circulation are coordinately regulated such that systemic glucose balance is maintained, hypoglycemia (as well as hyperglycemia) is prevented, and a continuous supply of glucose to the brain is ensured (Table 2.2).[3–6,39]

Glucose influx into the circulation is the sum of intermittent exogenous glucose delivery from ingested carbohydrates and regulated endogenous glucose production from the liver (glycogenolysis and gluconeogenesis) and the kidneys (gluconeogenesis). Glucose efflux out of the circulation is the sum of ongoing fixed glucose utilization, largely by the brain, but to a small extent by strictly glycolytic tissues, such as the renal medullae and erythrocytes, and regulated glucose utilization by insulin-sensitive tissues, such as muscle, fat, liver, and kidneys among others. Because exogenous glucose delivery is intermittent and much of glucose utilization (largely that by the brain) is fixed, the plasma glucose concentration is maintained and systemic glucose balance is fine-tuned by regulated endogenous glucose production and regulated glucose utilization by nonneural tissues.[3–6,39,40]

The liver is the major site of net endogenous glucose production, but net renal glucose production has been demonstrated under some conditions, including prolonged fasting and hypoglycemia, in humans.[41,42] Resumption of endogenous glucose production during the anhepatic phase of human liver transplantation,[43] documented extrahepatic glucose production, and data from a mouse model of inducible liver-specific deletion of the glucose-6-phosphatase gene have provided evidence of physiologically important extrahepatic glucose production.[44] In the mice, fasting plasma glucose concentrations fell initially but then became similar to those in control animals after ~30 h, a finding attributed by the authors to increased renal and intestinal glucose production.

Although an array of hormonal, neural, and substrate factors are involved, glucose production and utilization are regulated primarily by the pancreatic β-cell hormone insulin. As plasma glucose concentrations rise (e.g., after a meal), insulin secretion increases and both suppresses hepatic (and renal) glucose production and stimulates glucose utilization by muscle and fat. As plasma glucose concentrations decline (e.g., between meals), insulin secretion decreases and both increases hepatic (and renal) glucose production and decreases glucose utilization by muscle and fat. Importantly, although insulin acts throughout the brain[45]—both directly to decrease food intake, increase cognition, maintain body temperature, increase cholesterol biosynthesis, and

Table 2.2—Systemic Glucose Balance

Glucose flux into the circulation	Glucose flux out of the circulation
Intermittent exogenous glucose delivery	Ongoing glucose utilization, largely by the brain (plus strictly glycolytic tissues)
+	+
Regulated endogenous glucose production:	Regulated glucose utilization
• Liver: glycogenolysis and gluconeogenesis[a,c,d]	• Muscle, fat, liver, kidneys, etc.[b,e]
• Kidneys: gluconeogenesis[a,d]	

[a]Decreased by insulin; [b]increased by insulin; [c]increased by glucagon; [d]increased by epinephrine; [e]decreased by epinephrine.

maintain the sympathoadrenal response to hypoglycemia and via the brain to decrease hepatic glucose production, increase white fat lipogenesis, increase brown fat thermogenesis, maintain reproductive function, and increase sympathoadrenal activity—insulin does not stimulate blood-to-brain glucose transport.[46,47]

Insulin is a potent and critical hormone. Its deficiency causes hyperglycemia (diabetes), and its excess can cause hypoglycemia.[3–6,31,39,40] Nonetheless, it is not the only factor involved in the maintenance of systemic glucose balance. At the least, the plasma glucose–raising (glucose counterregulatory) hormones glucagon, epinephrine, cortisol, and growth hormone also are involved.

Glucoregulatory Factors

Insulin

Insulin secretion is stimulated by glucose, amino acids, nonesterified fatty acids, β_2-adrenergic activation by catecholamines such as epinephrine, acetylcholine released from parasympathetic nerves, glucagon-like peptide-1, and glucose-dependent insulinotropic polypeptide. It is inhibited by low glucose, α_2-adrenergic activation by catecholamines such as norepinephrine released from sympathetic nerves, and somatostatin. Insulin secretion is sensitive to fluctuations in the plasma glucose concentration within the physiological range (Table 2.1).[3–6,39,40,48]

Insulin is secreted from pancreatic islet β-cells into the hepatic portal vein. Approximately 50% is extracted by the liver.[40] Insulin secretion can be quantified by measurements of the plasma concentrations of C-peptide, the peptide cleaved from proinsulin to produce insulin.[49,50] C-peptide is co-secreted with insulin but is not cleared by the liver. Insulin secretion so calculated virtually ceases during hypoglycemia in humans.[48]

The physiology of insulin action has been reviewed.[51] Insulin suppresses hepatic glycogenolysis rapidly and hepatic (and renal) gluconeogenesis more gradually, and thus it suppresses endogenous glucose production.[3–6,39,40,52] Basal insulin levels restrain glucose production in the postabsorptive state, and increased insulin levels suppress glucose production and stimulate glucose utilization in the postprandial state. The actions of insulin to suppress glucose production are both direct (via hepatic and renal insulin receptors) and indirect.[3,4,6,39,40,52–55] The hormone acts indirectly by inhibition of lipolysis, suppression of glucagon secretion, limitation of gluconeogenic precursor (e.g., lactate, amino acids, glycerol) flux from muscle and fat to the liver (and kidneys), and CNS-mediated activation of parasympathetic outflow. Because insulin suppresses lipolysis and ketogenesis, stimulates glycolysis, and inhibits gluconeogenesis, serum-free (nonesterified) fatty acid and ketone body concentrations decrease and serum lactate concentrations increase during hyperinsulinemic euglycemic and hypoglycemic clamps.[56,57]

Conversely, a decrease in insulin, as during decreasing plasma glucose concentrations and hypoglycemia, causes an increase in hepatic (and renal) glucose production, an initial increase in hepatic glycogenolysis, and virtual cessation of glucose utilization by insulin-sensitive tissues.[3–6,39,40,48] As discussed later in this chapter, a decrease in insulin is the first physiological defense against hypoglycemia.[3,39]

Glucagon

The evolution of knowledge about glucagon has been summarized.[58] Glucagon secretion is stimulated by low glucose, amino acids, β_2-adrenergic activation by catecholamines such as epinephrine and norepinephrine, acetylcholine released from parasympathetic nerves, and glucose-dependent insulinotropic polypeptide. It is inhibited by high glucose, insulin, nonesterified fatty acids, somatostatin, and glucagon-like peptide-1.[3–6,39,40] Whereas it is less sensitive to decreasing glucose levels than insulin secretion, glucagon secretion increases as plasma glucose concentrations fall just below the physiological range(Table 2.1).[26–28]

A decrease in β-cell insulin secretion normally stimulates glucagon secretion during hypoglycemia.[56,57,59–64] That is made possible by the intimate relationship between β-cells and α-cells in human islets.[65] The regulation of glucagon secretion by nutrients, hormones, neurotransmitters, and drugs is complex and incompletely understood.[57,64] It involves direct signaling of α-cells,[66] indirect intraislet signaling of α-cells by β-cell secretory products including insulin[57] and the δ-cell secretory product somatostatin,[67] and indirect extra-islet signaling by the autonomic nervous system[68,69] and by gut incretins.[70] Among the intraislet factors, β-cell secretion appears to play an important role as selective destruction of β-cells in type 1 diabetes (T1D) results in the loss of the glucagon secretory response to hypoglycemia,[71] and partial reduction of β-cell mass in minipigs results in impaired postprandial suppression of glucagon secretion.[72] Glucagon secretion is not critically dependent on extra-islet signaling. Hypoglycemia increases glucagon secretion from the denervated (transplanted) human pancreas[73] and the denervated dog pancreas,[74] as well as in the spinal cord–transected human,[75] and the glucagon response is quantitatively normal. Furthermore, low glucose increases glucagon secretion from the perfused rodent pancreas[76] and perifused rodent and human islets, that is, in the absence of neural and gut factors. Evidence suggests that insulin restrains glucagon secretion partially through central actions as well as through direct α-cell actions.[77] But, again, glucagon secretion is not critically dependent on extra-islet signaling. The evidence that insulin reciprocally regulates glucagon secretion has been reviewed.[5,78]

Glucagon is secreted from pancreatic islet α-cells into the hepatic portal vein. Approximately 25% is extracted by the liver.[40] The hormone generally is thought to act only on the liver where it stimulates glucose production[79]; however, it is lipolytic in high doses. The absence of a marker of glucagon secretion (analogous to C-peptide for insulin secretion) complicates the assessment of glucagon secretion in humans. Furthermore, many glucagon immunoassays measure species in addition to biologically active 3,500-Dalton glucagon, although changes in measured glucagon levels are thought to reflect changes in biologically active glucagon.[40] In addition, because insulin suppresses glucagon secretion, the glucagon responses to hypoglycemia measured during contemporary hyperinsulinemic-hypoglycemic clamps are much less robust than the responses measured during hypoglycemia induced by an intravenous bolus injection of insulin.

Glucagon rapidly stimulates hepatic (but not renal) glucose production, largely by stimulating glycogenolysis.[3,4,39,40,79] The increases in glucose production and the plasma glucose concentration are transient, in part because of increased insulin secretion and the suppressive effect of hyperglycemia on glucose production.[40] Glucagon also stimulates hepatic gluconeogenesis when gluconeogenic precursors are abundant, as they are when epinephrine levels are also elevated.[80] The hepatic glycogenolytic response to glucagon is enhanced by nearly threefold during insulin-induced hypoglycemia.[81] The extent to which that increased sensitivity to glucagon over insulin is the result of a synergistic interaction between glucagon and other glucose-raising systems, such as the sympathoadrenal system, activated by hypoglycemia, by hypoglycemia per se, or both is not known.

Glucagon, in concert with insulin, supports the postabsorptive plasma glucose concentration in humans.[40,82,83] Indeed, glucagon likely plays a role in the pathogenesis of hyperglycemia in diabetes.[54,78,84,85] As discussed later in this chapter, an increase in glucagon is the second physiological defense against hypoglycemia.[3,39]

Epinephrine and the Sympathoadrenal System

The autonomic nervous system includes the sympathetic nervous system and the adrenal medullae, collectively termed the sympathoadrenal system, and the parasympathetic nervous system. All three components are involved in metabolic regulation, including glucoregulation[3–6,39]: sympathoadrenal activation raises plasma glucose concentrations and parasympathetic activation tends to lower plasma glucose concentrations. Postganglionic sympathetic neurons release norepinephrine or acetylcholine, and postganglionic parasympathetic neurons release acetylcholine, within innervated tissues. Whereas some extra-adrenal chromaffin cells persist into adult life, the major residual clusters of chromaffin cells make up the adrenal medullae, which are virtually the sole source of the circulating hormone epinephrine.[3–6,34,39] The anatomical relationship between the adrenal medullae and the adrenal cortices is important physiologically because a portal venous system provides cortisol from the cortex to the medulla, where the enzyme that catalyzes the conversion of norepinephrine to epinephrine (phenylethanolamine-*N*-methyltransferase) is cortisol induced.[86,87] Thus, adrenocortical cortisol deficiency results in adrenomedullary epinephrine deficiency,[87] including a markedly reduced plasma epinephrine response to hypoglycemia in humans.[88]

Unlike insulin and glucagon secretion, which are regulated primarily by changes in glucose concentrations within the pancreatic islets and only secondarily by autonomic mechanisms, sympathoadrenal activity, including epinephrine secretion, is regulated within the CNS.[3,39] For example, subphysiological plasma glucose concentrations, sensed in the periphery (e.g., in the portal and mesenteric veins) and in the CNS,[89–93] trigger a centrally mediated sympathoadrenal discharge—the magnitude of which is a function of the nadir glucose concentration—resulting in an increase in circulating epinephrine and norepinephrine. The epinephrine response is derived almost exclusively from the adrenal medullae.[34] Whereas circulating norepinephrine is largely derived from sympathetic nerves under resting and many stimulated (e.g., exercise) conditions,[94] the increment in plasma norepinephrine during hypoglycemia is largely derived from the adrenal medullae.[34]

The biochemistry and the integrated physiology of the human sympathoadrenal system have been reviewed in detail.[95] Epinephrine and norepinephrine are released from adrenomedullary chromaffin cells into the circulation; as such, these catecholamines function as classical hormones.[3,4,6,39] In addition, norepinephrine is released from axon terminals of sympathetic postganglionic neurons into synaptic clefts in direct relationship to adrenergic receptors on target cells and functions as a neurotransmitter.[3,4,6,39] Most of the neurally released norepinephrine is recaptured into axon terminals (or is metabolized locally); perhaps only 10% enters the circulation. Most metabolism of catecholamines occurs in the cytoplasm of the cells in which the amines are produced as a result of leakage from storage vesicles into the cytoplasm or during transit through the cytoplasm after reuptake from the extracellular space.[95] Sympathetic postganglionic neurons largely express the degradative enzyme monoamine oxidase and therefore produce deaminated metabolites of norepinephrine (e.g., 3,4-dihydroxyphenylglycol). However, adrenomedullary chromaffin cells also express the enzyme catechol-O-methyltransferase and primarily produce the 3-O-methyl metabolites of epinephrine and norepinephrine, metanephrine, and normetanephrine. In humans, >90% of circulating metanephrine, and ~33% of circulating normetanephrine, are derived from the adrenal medullae.[95] Thus, stimulated plasma metanephrine concentrations can be conceptualized as a measure of the adrenomedullary epinephrine secretory capacity.

Measurement of the plasma epinephrine concentration provides a useful index of adrenomedullary activity,[34] although, like that of other hormones, it represents the balance between secretion and clearance. The evaluation of sympathetic neural activity is more problematic. Although circulating norepinephrine is largely derived from adrenergic sympathetic postganglionic neurons under resting and many stimulated conditions,[94] the increase in plasma norepinephrine concentrations during hypoglycemia is largely derived from the adrenal medulla.[34] Furthermore, even under the appropriate conditions, circulating norepinephrine represents only a small fraction of that released from sympathetic nerves and is the net result of differentiated regional nerve firing. Isotope dilution estimates of systemic and regional norepinephrine spillover have been used to overcome these shortcomings[96,97] and have documented sympathetic neural responses to hypoglycemia, although the fundamental assumptions of the method have been questioned.[98] Microneurography measures muscle sympathetic nerve activity directly and has documented an increase in this nerve activity during hypoglycemia.[99,100] The method, however, is operator dependent, time-consuming, and demanding for the subject; does not allow movement by the subject; is not practical in the presence of autonomic neuropathy; and measures only one aspect of sympathetic nerve activity in only one region of the body (typically the lower extremity). Another approach is measurement of the extracellular norepinephrine concentration by microdialysis.[101,102] That method has been used to document norepinephrine release in skeletal muscle and fat during hypoglycemia.[102] It requires careful calibration and is applicable to limited regions of the body. Finally, as noted earlier, adrenergic and cholinergic symptoms[30] reflect the sympathetic neural response to hypoglycemia.[34]

Like glucagon, epinephrine rapidly stimulates hepatic glycogenolysis; it stimulates hepatic gluconeogenesis more prominently than glucagon.[80] Unlike glucagon, epinephrine also stimulates renal gluconeogenesis and glucose production,[42] limits glucose clearance by insulin-sensitive tissues such as muscle, mobilizes gluconeogenic precursors from muscle (lactate, amino acids) and fat (glycerol) to the liver and kidneys, and suppresses insulin secretion.[3,4,6,39,80,103,104]

The mechanisms of the plasma glucose–raising effect of epinephrine, summarized in Figure 2.2, are complex.[39,105] They involve both direct (on the liver and kidneys) and indirect (other hormone- or substrate-mediated) actions, include stimulation of glucose production and limitation of glucose utilization, and are mediated through both β- and α-adrenergic receptors. Whereas many of the actions of the hormone involve β_2-adrenergic receptors (Figure 2.2), β_2-adrenergic activation alone has little plasma glucose–raising effect in healthy individuals because it also stimulates insulin secretion. Thus, α_2-adrenergic limitation of insulin secretion is normally an important aspect of the glycemic effect of epinephrine. Nonetheless, there is normally a small increase in insulin secretion—in response to β_2-adrenergic β-cell stimulation, rising plasma glucose concentrations, or both—over time.[104] That, too, is a critical glucoregulatory event because it limits the magnitude of the glycemic response. The glycemic response to epinephrine is increased substantially when insulin secretion is held constant pharmacologically in healthy individuals and in patients with T1D who cannot increase insulin secretion.[104] As discussed later in this chapter, an increase in epinephrine is the third defense against hypoglycemia.

Similar mechanisms are thought to be involved in the glycemic response to sympathetic neural norepinephrine release.[3,4,6,39] The adrenergic and cholinergic neurogenic symptoms caused by the intense sympathoadrenal

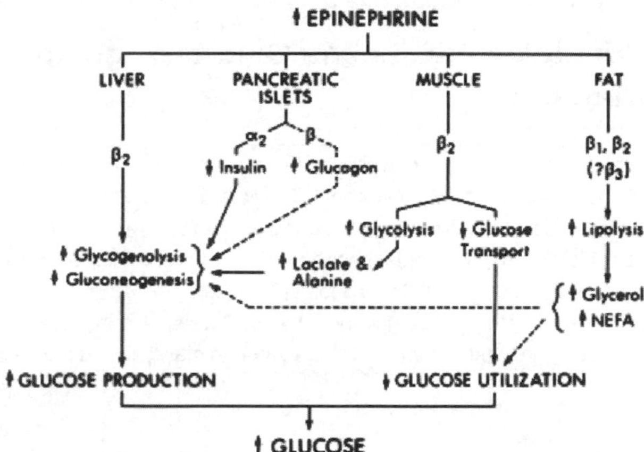

Figure 2.2—Mechanisms of the hyperglycemic effect of epinephrine. The α and β symbols refer to α-adrenergic β-adrenergic receptors.

Source: From Cryer[105] with permission from the American Diabetes Association.

response to frank hypoglycemia prompt awareness of hypoglycemia.[30,34] As discussed later in this chapter, that awareness prompts the behavioral defense against hypoglycemia, ingestion of carbohydrates.

Cortisol and Growth Hormone

The plasma glucose–raising actions of glucagon and epinephrine occur within minutes.[3,39,40] In contrast, those of cortisol[106] and growth hormone[107] (both of which support glucose production and limit glucose clearance) are delayed for several hours. Importantly, none of these hormones (glucagon, epinephrine, cortisol, or growth hormone) alters glucose transport across the blood-brain barrier.

Glucose Counterregulation: The Prevention and Correction of Hypoglycemia

Physiological Defenses

As reviewed in detail,[39] there are three principles for the physiological prevention or correction of hypoglycemia (Table 2.3).[108–111] First, the prevention and correction of hypoglycemia are the result of both waning of

Table 2.3—Principles of Glucose Counterregulation in Humans

1. The prevention and correction of hypoglycemia are the result of both waning of insulin and activation of glucose counterregulatory systems. They are not due solely to waning of insulin.
2. Whereas insulin is the dominant plasma glucose–lowering factor, there are redundant glucose counterregulatory factors. Those include other hormones as well as substrates and perhaps neural factors. These collectively constitute a fail-safe system.
3. There is a hierarchy among the glucoregulatory factors. Decrements in insulin, increments in glucagon, and, absent the latter, increments in epinephrine stand high in that hierarchy.

insulin and activation of glucose counterregulatory (plasma glucose–raising) systems. They are not due solely to waning of insulin. After intravenous insulin injection, the changes in glucose kinetics that ultimately restore euglycemia—an increase in insulin-suppressed glucose production and a decrease in insulin-stimulated glucose utilization—begin while plasma insulin concentrations are still tenfold above baseline and in temporal relation to increments in the plasma levels of counterregulatory hormones.[108,109] Similarly, the changes in glucose kinetics that limit the hypoglycemic response to prolonged hyperinsulinemia occur despite sustained hyperinsulinemia.[112] In addition, hypoinsulinemia is not critical to recovery from hypoglycemia.[48] Furthermore, when insulin levels are held constant, interruption of the secretion or actions of glucose counterregulatory factors impairs the prevention or correction of hypoglycemia (see the next section). Second, although insulin is the dominant plasma glucose–lowering factor, there are redundant glucose counterregulatory factors.[110,111] These collectively constitute a fail-safe system that prevents or minimizes failure of the glucose counterregulatory process upon failure of one, or perhaps more, of its components. Third, there is a hierarchy among the redundant glucoregulatory factors—that is, a ranked series of counterregulatory factors, some more critical to the effectiveness of the fail-safe system than others—that act in concert with decrements in insulin to prevent or correct hypoglycemia.[110,111] Several aspects of this physiology are also shown in Table 2.1. Studies of its mechanisms in humans are summarized in Figure 2.3[113] and Figure 2.4.[114]

In defense against falling plasma glucose concentrations, decrements in insulin are fundamentally important. Insulin secretion virtually ceases during hypoglycemia and increments in insulin from suppressed

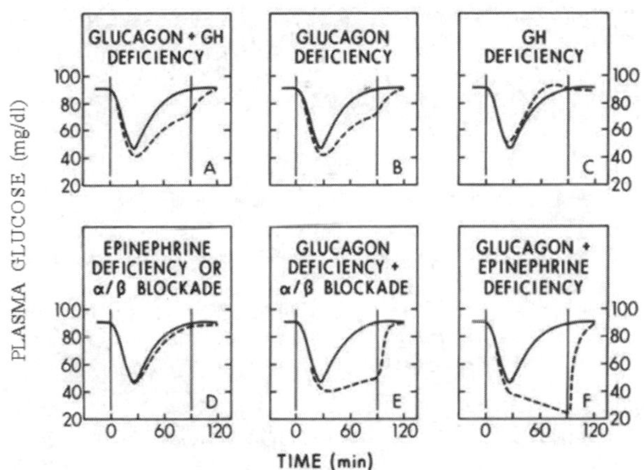

Figure 2.3—Summary of studies of the mechanisms of recovery from short-term hypoglycemia, induced by intravenous insulin injection at time 0 min, in humans. Interventions were started at time 0 min and stopped at 90 min (i.e., between the vertical lines in each panel). Plasma glucose curves in control studies are indicated by the solid lines (the same in all panels), and plasma glucose curves under the indicated conditions are shown by the dashed lines. GH, growth hormone.

Source: From Cryer[113] with permission from the American Diabetes Association.

levels impair recovery from hypoglycemia in a dose-related fashion.[48] An increase in insulin secretion is the first, and for practical purposes the only, defense against rising plasma glucose concentrations; loss of β-cell insulin secretion causes hyperglycemia (diabetes) and is fatal if insulin is not replaced. Conversely, a decrease in insulin secretion is the first, and arguably the most important, defense against falling plasma glucose concentrations. But, it is not the only defense. Glucose counterregulatory systems can prevent or correct hypoglycemia despite moderate hyperinsulinemia.

Among the glucose counterregulatory factors, glucagon plays a primary role.[110,111] Albeit demonstrably involved, epinephrine is not normally critical. But, it becomes critical when glucagon is deficient. Isolated deficiency of the glucagon response[115] or of epinephrine actions[116] result in lower nadir plasma

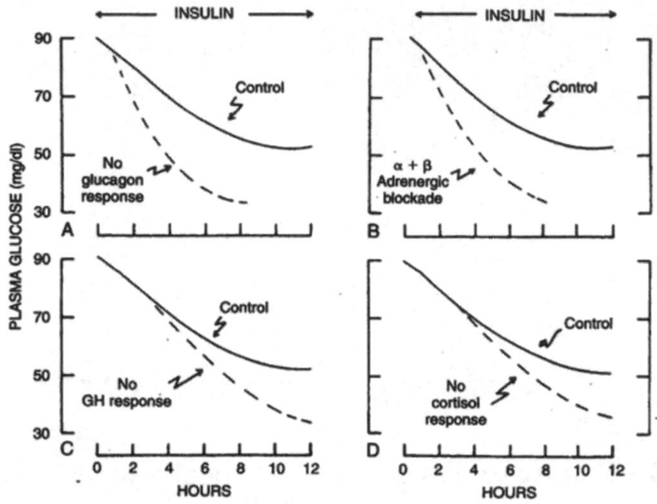

Figure 2.4—Summary of studies of the mechanisms of the defense against prolonged insulin-induced hypoglycemia in humans. Plasma glucose curves in control studies are indicated by the solid lines (the same in all panels), and plasma glucose curve, the indicated conditions are shown by the dashed lines.

Source: From Gerich[114] with permission from the American Diabetes Association.

glucose concentrations early in the course of prolonged hypoglycemia. These data document that both glucagon and epinephrine are involved in defense against hyperinsulinemia. They do not address the relative roles of glucagon or epinephrine in the prevention or correction of hypoglycemia. Suppression of glucagon secretion (with somatostatin) impairs, but does not prevent, recovery from short-term hypoglycemia.[110,111] That effect is reversed by glucagon, but not by growth hormone, replacement. In contrast, neither pharmacological adrenergic blockade nor epinephrine deficiency (bilateral adrenalectomy) impairs recovery from short-term hypoglycemia. Progressive hypoglycemia, however, develops when both glucagon and epinephrine are deficient. These data indicate that glucagon is involved in the correction of hypoglycemia, whereas epinephrine is not critical when glucagon secretion is intact. Epinephrine becomes critical when glucagon secretion is deficient. Suppression of glucagon secretion lowers plasma glucose concentrations after an overnight fast,[82,83,117] during a prolonged fast,[118] late after glucose ingestion,[119,120] and during moderate exercise.[121,122] In contrast, with the exception of a small effect during exercise, neither pharmacological adrenergic blockade nor epinephrine deficiency lowers plasma glucose concentrations under any of these conditions.[117–122] Combined glucagon deficiency and adrenergic blockade (or epinephrine deficiency), however, results in progressive hypoglycemia under all four conditions.[117–122] These data further indicate that glucagon plays a role in the prevention and correction of hypoglycemia under diverse physiological conditions, whereas epinephrine is not critical when glucagon secretion is intact. Epinephrine becomes critical to the prevention or correction of hypoglycemia under diverse conditions when glucagon secretion is deficient. The role of glucagon in the pathogenesis of hypoglycemia (and hyperglycemia) in diabetes has been reviewed.[5,78]

Growth hormone and cortisol stand lower in the hierarchy of physiological glucose counterregulatory factors than insulin, glucagon, and epinephrine.[123–125] Both growth hormone[123] and cortisol[124] are involved in defense against prolonged hypoglycemia, but neither is critical to the correction of even prolonged hypoglycemia or the prevention of hypoglycemia after an overnight fast.[125]

Evidence indicates that glucose autoregulation—an increase in endogenous glucose production independent of hormonal and neural regulatory signals—is involved in glucose counterregulation, albeit only during severe hypoglycemia,[126] and that nonesterified fatty acids mediate, at least in part, the glucose counterregulatory actions of epinephrine.[127]

Evidence is unclear whether efferent neural mechanisms normally play an important role in physiological glucose counterregulation. Sympathoadrenal activation, however, does play a key role in the behavioral defense against developing hypoglycemia.

Behavioral Defense

If the physiological defenses fail to reverse falling plasma glucose concentrations, lower plasma glucose levels trigger a more intense sympathoadrenal response, which causes symptoms[30,34] that allow the individual to recognize hypoglycemia. Again, the neurogenic symptoms of hypoglycemia are largely the result of sympathetic neural, rather than adrenomedullary, activation.[34] That awareness of hypoglycemia prompts the behavioral defense against hypoglycemia, ingestion of carbohydrates.

Integrated Physiology of Glucose Counterregulation

The integrated physiology of glucose counterregulation—the mechanisms that normally prevent or rapidly correct hypoglycemia in humans[39]—is summarized in Figure 2.5.[128] The first defense against falling plasma glucose concentrations is a decrease in pancreatic β-cell insulin secretion. The second defense is an increase in pancreatic α-cell glucagon secretion. The third defense, which becomes critical when glucagon is deficient, is an increase in adrenomedullary epinephrine secretion. If these three physiological defenses fail to abort the episode, lower plasma glucose

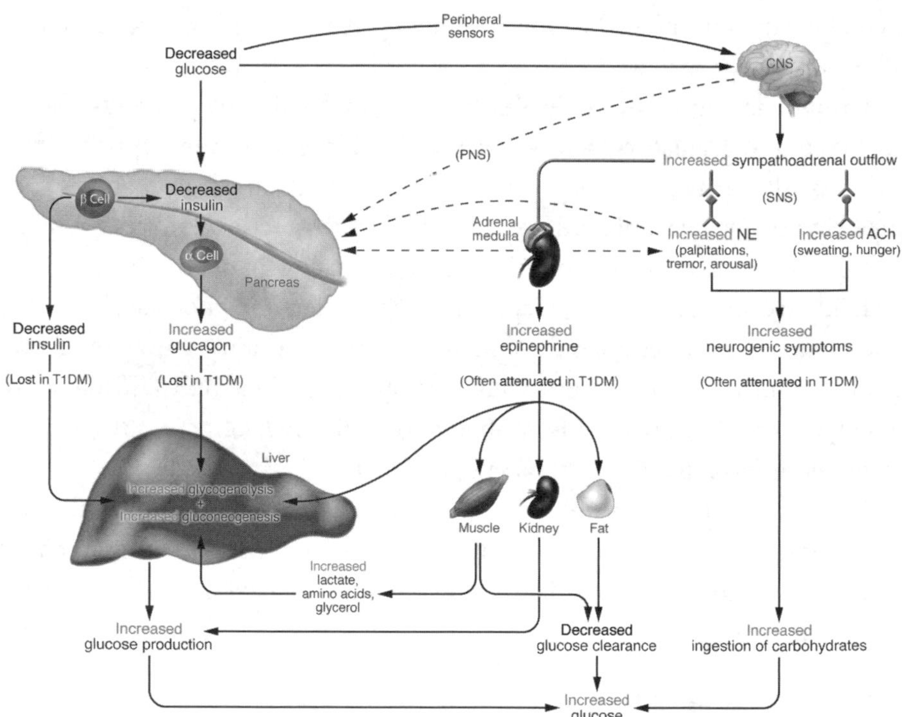

Figure 2.5—Physiological and behavioral defenses against hypoglycemia in humans. Ach, acetylcholine, NE, norepinephrine; PNS, parasympathetic nervous system; sympathetic nervous system; T1D, type 1 diabetes.

Source: From Cryer[128] 2006 with permission from the American Society for Clinical Investigation.

levels trigger a more intense sympathoadrenal (sympathetic neural as well as adrenomedullary) response that causes symptoms and thus triggers awareness of hypoglycemia prompting the behavioral defense.

The mechanisms of the normal responses to falling plasma glucose concentrations (Figure 2.5) are further illustrated in Figure 2.6. Low plasma glucose concentrations are sensed by pancreatic β-cells, resulting in a decrease in insulin secretion. The resulting decrease in intraislet insulin, perhaps among other β-cell secretory products, in concert with low glucose levels, signals an increase in α-cell glucagon secretion.[5,56,57,64,78] Thus, the first and second physiological defenses against falling plasma glucose concentrations—a decrement in insulin secretion and an increment in glucagon secretion—are mediated at the level of the pancreatic islets. CNS connections (i.e., innervation) are not required. Because appropriate changes in insulin and glucagon secretion are sufficient to defend against falling plasma glucose concentrations, the CNS is not normally critical to the prevention or correction of hypoglycemia. It becomes critical, however, when the appropriate insulin and glucagon responses do not occur (see Chapter 3).

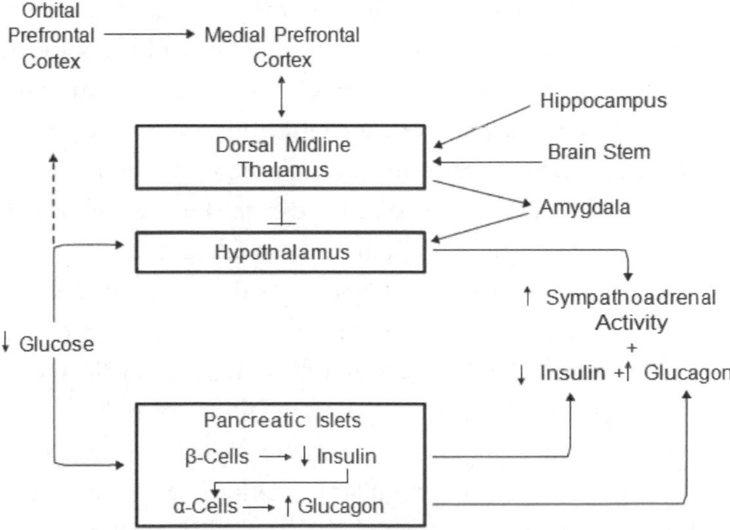

Figure 2.6—Schematic representation of the normal pancreatic, hypothalamic, and cerebral mechanisms of the glucose counterregulatory responses to falling plasma glucose concentrations in humans.

Low plasma glucose concentrations are sensed in peripheral sites (such as the hepatic portal or mesenteric vein as well as the gut, carotid, body, and oral cavity) and are transmitted to the brain and also are sensed directly within the brain.[69,129] There, the hypothalamus initiates an increase in systemic sympathoadrenal activity, including the third physiological defense against falling plasma glucose concentrations—an increment in adrenomedullary epinephrine secretion. That increase in sympathoadrenal activity also includes activation of the sympathetic nervous system and thus, ultimately, the behavioral defense against falling plasma glucose concentrations (the ingestion of carbohydrates). Although sympathoadrenal activation tends to decrease insulin secretion and increase glucagon secretion, those insulin and glucagon responses do not require a sympathoadrenal response, because they also are signaled at the level of the pancreatic islets.[56,57,78]

Evidence is increasing that the hypothalamic response is modulated by widespread functionally interconnected cerebral inputs,[130–132] including an inhibitory pathway from the dorsal midline thalamus (Figure 2.6). The details of hypothalamic and cerebral mechanisms remain to be determined, however.[69,90,133]

At least in part because of the clinical importance of hypoglycemia in people with diabetes, studies of the molecular and cellular physiology and pathophysiology of the CNS-mediated neuroendocrine, including sympathoadrenal, responses to falling plasma glucose concentrations are an increasingly active area of fundamental neuroscience research. Some of these mechanisms have been reviewed,[5,69,90,133] and these are discussed in the context of the pathophysiology of glucose counterregulation in diabetes in Chapter 3.

Interestingly, there is only one physiologically effective defense against hyperglycemia, the glucoregulatory hormone insulin, whereas there are redundant physiological and behavioral defenses against hypoglycemia. This may explain why glucoregulatory failure resulting from relative or absolute insulin deficiency causing hyperglycemia (diabetes) is common, whereas glucose counterregulatory failure causing hypoglycemia is rare in the absence of drug-treated diabetes. This dichotomy is plausibly explained by evolutionary pressure. Typically developing later in life, diabetes would have threatened survival of the individual. In contrast, hypoglycemia would have threatened survival of the species. The irony is that in the setting of demonstrably effective insulin secretagogue or insulin therapy of diabetes, the causative β-cell failure also leads to compromised physiological and behavioral defenses against hypoglycemia (see Chapter 3).

References

1. Clarke DD, Sokoloff L. Circulation and energy metabolism of the brain. In *Basic Neurochemistry: Molecular, Cellular and Medical Aspects.* 5th ed. Siegel G, Agranoff B, Albers RW, Molinoff P, Eds. New York, Raven Press, 1994, p. 645–680
2. Cryer PE. Hypoglycemia, functional brain failure, and brain death. *J Clin Invest* 2007;117:868–870
3. Cryer PE. The barrier of hypoglycemia in diabetes. *Diabetes* 2008;57:3169–3176
4. Cryer PE. Hypoglycemia in diabetes. In *Textbook of Diabetes.* 4th ed. Holt RIG, Cockram C, Flyvbjerg A, Goldstein BJ, Eds. Oxford, U.K., Wiley-Blackwell, 2010, p. 528–545
5. Cryer PE. Mechanisms of hypoglycemia-associated autonomic failure in diabetes. *N Engl J Med* 2013;369:362–372
6. Cryer PE. Hypoglycemia. In *Williams Textbook of Endocrinology*. 13th ed. Melmed S, Polonsky KS, Larsen PR, Kronenberg HM, Eds. Philadelphia, Elsevier, 2016, p. 1582–1607
7. Itoh Y, Esaki T, Shimoji K, Cook M, Law MJ, Kaufman E, Sokoloff L. Dichloroacetate effects on glucose and lactate oxidation by neurons and astroglia in vitro and on glucose utilization by brain in vivo. *Proc Natl Acad Sci USA* 2003;100:4879–4884
8. Hyder F, Patel AB, Gjedde A, Rothman DL, Behar KL, Shulman RG. Neuronal-glial glucose oxidation and glutaminergic-GABAergic function. *J Cerebr Blood Flow Metab* 2006;26:865–877
9. Magistretti, PJ. Neuron-glia metabolic coupling and plasticity. *J Exp Biol* 2006;209:2304–2311
10. Owen OE, Felig P, Morgan AP, Wahren J, Cahill GF. Liver and kidney metabolism during prolonged starvation. *J Clin Invest* 1969;48:574–583
11. Nehlig A. Brain uptake and metabolism of ketone bodies in animal models. *Prostaglandins Leukot Essent Fatty Acids* 2004;70:265–275
12. Dalsgaard MK. Fuelling cerebral activity in exercising man. *J Cerebral Blood Flow Metab* 2006;26:731–750

13. Won SJ, Jang BG, Yoo BH, Sohn M, Lee MW, Choi BY, Kim JH, Song HK, Suh SW. Prevention of acute/severe hypoglycemia-induced neuron death by lactate administration. *J Cereb Blood Flow Metab* 2012;32:1086–1096

14. Fanelli CG, Paramore DS, Hershey T, Terkamp C, Ovalle F, Craft S, Cryer PE. Impact of nocturnal hypoglycemia on hypoglycemic cognitive dysfunction in type 1 diabetes. *Diabetes* 1998;47:1920–1927

15. Segel SA, Fanelli CG, Dence CS, Markham J, Videen TO, Paramore DS, Powers WJ, Cryer PE. Blood-to-brain glucose transport, cerebral glucose metabolism and cerebral blood flow are not increased following hypoglycemia. *Diabetes* 2001;50:1911–1917

16. van de Ven KCC, de Galan BE, van der Graaf M, Shestov AA, Henry P-G, Tack CJJ, Heerschap A. Effect of acute hypoglycemia on human cerebral glucose metabolism measured by ^{13}C magnetic resonance spectroscopy. *Diabetes* 2011;60:1467–1473

17. van de Ven KC, van der Graaf M, Tack CJ, Heerschap A, de Galan BE. Steady-state brain glucose concentrations during hypoglycemia in healthy humans and patients with type 1 diabetes. *Diabetes* 2012;61:1974–1977

18. Antenor-Dorsey JAV, Khoury N, Su Y, Shackleford AM, Jethi KG, Powers WJ, Cryer PE, Arbeláez AM. The adrenomedullary epinephrine response to declining plasma glucose concentrations is a signaling event that is not caused by a decrease in the cerebral metabolic rate of glucose (abstract). *Diabetes* 2013; 62:A100

19. Wahren J, Ekberg K, Fernqvist-Forbes E, Nair S. Brain substrate utilization during acute hypoglycaemia. *Diabetologia* 1999;42:812–818

20. Lubow JM, Piñón IG, Avogaro A, Cobelli C, Treeson DM, Mandeville KA, Toffolo G, Boyle PJ. Brain oxygen utilization is unchanged by hypoglycemia in normal humans: lactate, alanine, and leucine uptake are not sufficient to offset energy deficit. *Am J Physiol Endocrinol Metab* 2006;290:E149–E153

21. Boumezbeur F, Petersen KF, Cline GW, Mason GF, Behar KL, Shulman GI, Rothman DL. The contribution of blood lactate to brain energy metabolism in humans measured by dynamic ^{13}C nuclear magnetic resonance spectroscopy. *J Neurosci* 2010;30:13983–13991

22. van Hall G, Strømstad M, Rasmussen P, Jans Ø, Zaar M, Gam C, Quistorff B, Secher NH, Nielsen HB. Blood lactate is an important energy source for the human brain. *J Cereb Blood Flow Metab* 2009;29:1121–1129

23. Herzog RI, Sherwin RS, Rothman DL. Insulin-induced hypoglycemia and its effect on the brain. Unraveling metabolism by in vivo nuclear magnetic resonance. *Diabetes* 2011;60:1856–1858

24. Öz G, Seaquist ER, Kumar A, Criego AB, Benedict LE, Rao JP, Henry P-G, Van De Moortele P-F, Gruetter R. Human brain glycogen content and metabolism: implications on its role in brain energy metabolism. *Am J Physiol Endocrinol Metab* 2007;292:E946–E951

25. Brown AM, Sickmann HM, Fosgerau K, Lund TM, Schousboe A, Waagepetersen HS, Ransom BR. Astrocyte glycogen metabolism is required for neural activity during aglycemia or intense stimulation in mouse white matter. *J Neurosci Res* 2005;79:74–80

26. Schwartz NS, Clutter WE, Shah SD, Cryer PE. Glycemic thresholds for activation of glucose counterregulatory systems are higher than the threshold for symptoms. *J Clin Invest* 1987;79:777–781

27. Mitrakou A, Ryan C, Veneman T, Mokan M, Jenssen T, Kiss I, Durrant J, Cryer P, Gerich J. Hierarchy of glycemic thresholds for counterregulatory hormone secretion, symptoms and cerebral dysfunction. *Am J Physiol Endocrinol Metab* 1991;260:E67–E74

28. Fanelli C, Pampanelli S, Epifano L, Rambotti AM, Ciofetta M, Modarelli F, Di Vincenzo A, Annibale B, Lepore M, Lalli C, Del Sindaco P, Brunetti P, Bolli GB. Relative roles of insulin and hypoglycaemia on induction of neuroendocrine responses to, symptoms of, and deterioration of cognitive function in hypoglycaemia in male and female humans. *Diabetologia* 1994;37:797–807

29. Cryer PE. Glycemic goals in diabetes: trade-off between glycemic control and iatrogenic hypoglycemia. *Diabetes* 2014;63:2188–2195

30. Towler DA, Havlin CE, Craft S, Cryer PE. Mechanism of awareness of hypoglycemia: perception of neurogenic (predominantly cholinergic) rather than neuroglycopenic symptoms. *Diabetes* 1993;42:1791–1798

31. Whipple AO. The surgical therapy of hyperinsulinism. *J Int Chir* 1938;3:237–276

32. Cryer PE, Axelrod L, Grossman AB, Heller SR, Montori VM, Seaquist ER, Service FJ. Evaluation and management of adult hypoglycemic disorders. *J Clin Endocrinol Metab* 2009;94:709–728

33. Deary IJ, Hepburn DA, MacLeod KM, Frier BM. Partitioning of the symptoms of hypoglycaemia using multi-sample confirmatory factor analysis. *Diabetologia* 1993;36:771–777

34. DeRosa MA, Cryer PE. Hypoglycemia and the sympathoadrenal system: neurogenic symptoms are largely the result of sympathetic neural, rather than adrenomedullary, activation. *Am J Physiol Endocrinol Metab* 2004;287:E32–E41

35. Schultes B, Jauch-Chara K, Gais S, Hallschmid M, Reiprich E, Kern W, Oltmanns KM, Peters A, Fehm HL, Born J. Defective awakening response to nocturnal hypoglycemia in patients with type 1 diabetes mellitus. *PLoS Medicine* 2007;4:e69

36. Sejling AS, Kjaer TW, Pedersen-Bjergaard U, Diemar SS, Frandsen CS, Hilsted L, Faber J, Holst JJ, Tarnow L, Nielsen MN, Remvig LS, Thorsteinsson B, Juhl CB. Hypoglycemia-associated changes in the electroencephalogram in patients with type 1 diabetes and normal hypoglycemia awareness or unawareness. *Diabetes* 2015;64:1760–1769

37. McCrimmon RJ, Deary IJ, Gold AE, Hepburn DA, MacLeod KM, Ewing FM, Frier BM. Symptoms reported during experimental hypoglycaemia: effect of method of induction of hypoglycaemia and of diabetes *per se*. *Diabet Med* 2003;20:507–509

38. Cox DJ, Gonder-Frederick L, Antoun B, Cryer PE, Clarke WL. Perceived symptoms in the recognition of hypoglycemia. *Diabetes Care* 1993;16:519–527

39. Cryer PE. The prevention and correction of hypoglycemia. In *Handbook of Physiology.* Section 7, The Endocrine System. Vol. II, The Endocrine Pancreas and Regulation of Metabolism. Jefferson LS, Cherrington AD, Eds. New York, Oxford University Press, 2001, p. 1057–1092

40. Cherrington AD. Control of glucose production in vivo by insulin and glucagon. In *Handbook of Physiology.* Section 7, The Endocrine System, Vol. II, The Endocrine Pancreas and Regulation of Metabolism. Jefferson LS, Cherrington AD, Eds. New York, Oxford University Press, 2001, p. 759–785

41. Gerich JE, Meyer C, Woerle HJ, Stumvoll M. Renal gluconeogenesis. *Diabetes Care* 2001;24:382–391

42. Gerich JE. Role of the kidney in normal glucose homeostasis and in the hyperglycaemia of diabetes mellitus: therapeutic implications. *Diabet Med* 2010;27:136–142

43. Joseph SE, Heaton N, Potter D, Pernet A, Umpleby MA, Amiel SA. Renal glucose production compensates for the liver during the anhepatic phase of liver transplantation. *Diabetes* 2000;49:450–456

44. Mutel E, Gautier-Stein A, Abdul-Wahed A, Amigó-Correig M, Zitoun C, Stefanutti A, Houberdon I, Tourette JA, Mithieux G, Rajas F. Control of blood glucose

in the absence of hepatic glucose production during prolonged fasting in mice. *Diabetes* 2011;60:3121–3131

45. Kleinridders A, Ferris HA, Cai W, Kahn CR. Insulin action in brain regulates systemic metabolism and brain function. *Diabetes* 2014;63:2232–2243

46. Knudsen GM, Hasselbach SG, Hertz MM, Paulson OB. High dose insulin does not increase glucose transfer across the blood-brain barrier in humans: a re-evaluation. *Eur J Clin Invest* 1999;29:687–691

47. Seaquist ER, Damberg GS, Tkac I, Gruetter R. The effect of insulin on in vivo cerebral glucose concentrations and rates of glucose transport/metabolism in humans. *Diabetes* 2001;50:2203–2209

48. Heller SR, Cryer PE. Hypoinsulinemia is not critical to glucose recovery from hypoglycemia in humans. *Am J Physiol Endocrinol Metab* 1991;261:E41–E48

49. Eaton RP, Allen RC, Schade DS, Erickson KM, Standefer J. Prehepatic insulin production in man: kinetic analysis using peripheral connecting peptide behavior. *J Clin Endocrinol Metab* 1980;51:520–528

50. Polonsky KS, Licinio-Paixao J, Given BD, Pugh W, Rue P, Galloway J, Karrison T, Frank B. Use of biosynthetic human C-peptide in the measurement of insulin secretion rates in normal volunteers and type I diabetic patients. *J Clin Invest* 1986;77:98–105

51. Ferrannini E. Physiology of glucose homeostasis and insulin therapy in type 1 and type 2 diabetes. *Endocrinol Metab Clin N Am* 2012;41:25–39

52. Edgerton DS, Lautz M, Scott M, Everett CA, Stettler KM, Neal DW, Chu CA, Cherrington AD. Insulin's direct effects on the liver dominate the control of hepatic glucose production. *J Clin Invest* 2006;116:521–527

53. Obici S, Zhang BB, Karkanias G, Rossetti L. Hypothalamic insulin signaling is required for inhibition of glucose production. *Nat Med* 2002;8:1376–1382

54. Edgerton DS, Cherrington AD. Glucagon as a critical factor in the pathology of diabetes. *Diabetes* 2011;60:377–380

55. Bergman RN. Orchestration of glucose homeostasis. *Diabetes* 2007;56:1489–1501

56. Raju B, Cryer PE. Loss of the decrement in intraislet insulin plausibly explains loss of the glucagon response to hypoglycemia in insulin-deficient diabetes. *Diabetes* 2005;54:757–764

57. Cooperberg BA, Cryer PE. Insulin reciprocally regulates glucagon secretion in humans. *Diabetes* 2010;59:2936–2940

58. Ahrén B. Glucagon–Early breakthroughs and recent discoveries. *Peptides* 2015;67:74–81

59. Maruyama H, Hisatomi A, Orci L, Grodsky GM, Unger RH. Insulin within islets is a physiologic glucagon release inhibitor. *J Clin Invest* 1984;74:2296–2299

60. Samols E, Stagner JI, Ewart RBL, Marks V. The order of islet microvascular cellular perfusion is B–A–D in the perfused rat pancreas. *J Clin Invest* 1988; 82:350–353

61. Banarer S, McGregor VP, Cryer PE. Intraislet hyperinsulinemia prevents the glucagon response to hypoglycemia despite an intact autonomic response. *Diabetes* 2002;51:958–965

62. Gosmanov NR, Szoke E, Israelian Z, Smith T, Cryer PE, Gerich JE, Meyer C. Role of the decrement in intraislet insulin for the glucagon response to hypoglycemia in humans. *Diabetes Care* 2005;28:1124–1131

63. Israelian Z, Gosmanov NR, Szoke E, Schorr M, Bokhari S, Cryer PE, Gerich JE, Meyer C. Increasing the decrement in intraislet insulin improves glucagon responses to hypoglycemia in advanced type 2 diabetes. *Diabetes Care* 2005;28:2691–2696

64. Cooperberg BA, Cryer PE. β-cell-mediated signaling predominates over direct α-cell signaling in the regulation of glucagon secretion in humans. *Diabetes Care* 2009;32:2275–2280

65. Bosco D, Armanet M, Morel P, Niclauss N, Sgroi A, Muller YD, Giovannoni L, Parnaud G, Berney T. Unique arrangement of alpha- and beta-cells in human islets of Langerhans. *Diabetes* 2010;59:1202–1210

66. Walker JN, Ramracheya R, Zhang Q, Johnson PRV, Braun M, Rorsman P. Regulation of glucagon secretion by glucose: paracrine, intrinsic or both? *Diabetes Obes Metab* 2011;13(Suppl. 1):95–105

67. Hauge-Evans AC, King AJ, Carmignac D, Richardson CC, Robinson ICAF, Low MJ, Christie MR, Persaud SJ, Jones PM. Somatostatin secreted by islet δ-cells fulfills multiple roles as a paracrine regulator of islet function. *Diabetes* 2009;58:403–411

68. Taborsky GJ Jr, Ahrén B, Havel PJ. Autonomic mediation of glucagon secretion during hypoglycemia. *Diabetes* 1998;47:995–1005

69. Marty N, Dallaporta M, Thorens B. Brain glucose sensing, counterregulation and energy homeostasis. *Physiology* 2007;22:241–251

70. Holst JJ. The physiology of glucagon-like peptide 1. *Physiol Rev* 2007;87: 1409–1439

71. Gerich JE, Langlois M, Noacco C, Karam J, Forsham P. Lack of glucagon response to hypoglycemia in diabetes: evidence for an intrinsic pancreatic alpha-cell defect. *Science* 1973;182:171–173

72. Meier JJ, Kjems LL, Veldhuis JD, Lefèbvre P, Butler PC. Postprandial suppression of glucagon secretion depends on intact pulsatile insulin secretion: further evidence for the intraislet insulin hypothesis. *Diabetes* 2006;55:1051–1056

73. Diem P, Redmon JB, Abid M, Moran A, Sutherland DER, Halter JB, Robertson RP. Glucagon, catecholamine and pancreatic polypeptide secretion in type 1 diabetic recipients of pancreatic allografts. *J Clin Invest* 1990;86:2008–2013

74. Sherck SM, Shiota M, Saccomando J, Cardin S, Allen EJ, Hastings JR, Neal DW, Williams PE, Cherrington AD. Pancreatic response to mild non-insulin induced hypoglycemia does not involve extrinsic neural input. *Diabetes* 2001;50:2487–2496

75. Palmer JP, Henry DP, Benson JW, Johnson DG, Ensinck JW. Glucagon response to hypoglycemia in sympathectomized man. *J Clin Invest* 1976;57:522–525

76. Gerich JE, Charles MA, Grodsky GM. Characterization of the effects of arginine and glucose on glucagon and insulin release from the perfused rat pancreas. *J Clin Invest* 1974;54:833–841

77. Paranjape SA, Chan O, Zhu W, Horblitt AM, McNay EC, Cresswell JA, Bogan JS, McCrimmon RJ, Sherwin RS. Influence of insulin in the ventromedial hypothalamus on pancreatic glucagon secretion in vivo. *Diabetes* 2010;59:1521–1527

78. Cryer PE. Glucagon in the pathogenesis of hypoglycemia and hyperglycemia in diabetes. *Endocrinology* 2012;153:1039–1048

79. Ramnanan CJ, Edgerton DS, Kraft G, Cherrington AD. Physiologic action of glucagon on liver glucose metabolism. *Diabetes Obes Metab* 2011;13(Suppl. 1): 118–125

80. Gustavson SM, Chu SA, Nishizawa M, Farmer B, Neal D, Yang Y, Vaughan S, Donahue EP, Flakoll P, Cherrington AD. Glucagon's actions are modified by the combination of epinephrine and gluconeogenic precursor infusion. *Am J Physiol Endocrinol Metab* 2003;285:E534–E544

81. Rivera N, Ramnanan CJ, An Z, Farmer T, Smith M, Farmer B, Irimia JM, Snead W, Lautz M, Roach PJ, Cherrington AD. Insulin-induced hypoglycemia increases hepatic sensitivity to glucagon in dogs. *J Clin Invest* 2010;120:4425–4435

82. Breckenridge SM, Cooperberg BA, Arbeláez AM, Patterson BW, Cryer PE. Glucagon, in concert with insulin, supports the postabsorptive plasma glucose concentration in humans. *Diabetes* 2007;56:2442–2448

83. Cooperberg BA, Cryer PE. Glucagon supports postabsorptive plasma glucose concentrations in humans with biologically optimal insulin levels. *Diabetes* 2010;59:2941–2944

84. Unger RH, Orci L. The essential role of glucagon in the pathogenesis of diabetes mellitus. *Lancet* 1975;1:14–16

85. Lee Y, Wang M-Y, Du XQ, Charron MJ, Unger RH. Glucagon receptor knockout prevents insulin-deficient type 1 diabetes in mice. *Diabetes* 2011;60:391–397

86. Wurtman RJ, Axelrod J. Adrenaline synthesis: control by the pituitary gland and adrenal glucocorticoids. *Science* 1965;150:1464–1465

87. Wurtman RJ. Stress and the adrenocortical control of epinephrine synthesis. *Metabolism* 2002;51:11–14

88. Davis SN, Shavers C, Davis B, Costa F. Prevention of an increase in plasma cortisol during hypoglycemia preserves subsequent counterregulatory responses. *J Clin Invest* 1997;100:429–438

89. Levin BE, Becker TC, Eiki J, Zhang BB, Dunn-Meynell AA. Ventromedial hypothalamic glucokinase is an important mediator of the counterregulatory response to insulin-induced hypoglycemia. *Diabetes* 2008;57:1371–1379

90. McCrimmon RY, Sherwin RS. Hypoglycemia in type 1 diabetes. *Diabetes* 2010;59:2333–2339

91. Levin BE, Magnan C, Dunn-Meynell A, Le Foll C. Metabolic sensing and the brain: who, what, where, and how? *Endocrinology* 2011;152:2552–2557

92. Jokiaho AJ, Donovan CM, Watts AG. The rate of fall of blood glucose determines the necessity of forebrain-projecting catecholaminergic neurons for male rat sympathoadrenal responses. *Diabetes* 2014;63:2854–2865

93. Bohland M, Matveyenk AV, Saberi M, Khan AM, Watts Ag, Donovan CM. Activation of hindbrain neurons is mediated by portal-mesenteric vein glucosensors during slow-onset hypoglycemia. *Diabetes* 2014;63:2866–2875

94. Goldstein DS, Kopin IJ. Adrenomedullary, adrenocortical, and sympathoneural responses to stressors: a metaanalysis. *Endocr Regul* 2008;42:111–119

95. Eisenhofer G, Kopin IJ, Goldstein DS. Catecholamine metabolism: a contemporary view with implications for physiology and medicine. *Pharmacological Reviews* 2004;56:331–349

96. Eisenhofer G. Sympathetic nerve function: assessment of radioisotope dilution analysis. *Clin Auton Res* 2005;15:264–283

97. Paramore DS, Fanelli CG, Shah SD, Cryer PE. Forearm norepinephrine spillover during standing, hyperinsulinemia and hypoglycemia. *Am J Physiol Endocrinol Metab* 1998;275:E872–E881

98. Christensen NJ, Norsk P. The fallacy of plasma noradrenaline spillover measurements. *Acta Physiol Scand* 2005;183:333–334

99. Vallbo AB, Hagbarth K-E, Wallin BG. Microneurography: how the technique developed and its role in the investigation of the sympathetic nervous system. *J Appl Physiol* 2004;96:1262–1269

100. Fagius J. Sympathetic nerve activity in metabolic control: some basic concepts. *Acta Physiol Scand* 2003;177:337–343

101. Bruce S, Tack C, Patel J, Pacak K, Goldstein DS. Local sympathetic function in human skeletal muscle and adipose tissue assessed by microdialysis. *Clin Auton Res* 2002;12:13–19

102. Maggs DG, Jacob R, Rife F, Caprio S, Tamborlane WV, Sherwin RS. Counterregulation in peripheral tissues. *Diabetes* 1997;46:70–76

103. Rizza RA, Cryer PE, Haymond MW, Gerich JE. Adrenergic mechanisms for the effect of epinephrine on glucose production and clearance in man. *J Clin Invest* 1980;65:682–689

104. Berk MA, Clutter WE, Skor D, Shah SD, Gingerich RP, Parvin CA, Cryer PE. Enhanced glycemic responsiveness to epinephrine in insulin-dependent diabetes mellitus is the result of the inability to secrete insulin. *J Clin Invest* 1985;75:1842–1851

105. Cryer PE. Catecholamines, pheochromocytoma and diabetes. *Diabetes Reviews* 1993;1:309–317

106. Rizza RA, Mandarino L, Gerich J. Cortisol-induced insulin resistance in man: impaired suppression of glucose production and stimulation of glucose utilization due to a post-receptor defect of insulin action. *J Clin Endocrinol Metab* 1982;54:131–138

107. MacGorman LR, Rizza RA, Gerich JE. Physiological concentrations of growth hormone exert insulin-like and insulin antagonistic effects on both hepatic and extrahepatic tissues in man. *J Clin Endocrinol Metab* 1981;53:556–559

108. Garber AJ, Cryer PE, Santiago JV, Haymond MW, Pagliara AS, Kipnis DM. The role of adrenergic mechanisms in the substrate and hormonal response to insulin-induced hypoglycemia in man. *J Clin Invest* 1976;58:7–15

109. Clarke WL, Santiago JV, Thomas L, Ben-Galim E, Haymond MW, Cryer PE. Adrenergic mechanisms in recovery from hypoglycemia in man: adrenergic blockade. *Am J Physiol Endocrinol Metab* 1979;236:E147–E152

110. Gerich J, Davis J, Lorenzi M, Rizza R, Bohannon N, Karam J, Lewis S, Kaplan R, Schultz T, Cryer P. Hormonal mechanisms of recovery from insulin-induced hypoglycemia in man. *Am J Physiol Endocrinol Metab* 1979;236:E380–E385

111. Rizza RA, Cryer PE, Gerich JE. Role of glucagon, catecholamines, and growth hormone in human glucose counterregulation. *J Clin Invest* 1979;64:62–71

112. De Feo P, Perriello G, De Cosmo S, Ventura MM, Campbell PJ, Brunetti P, Gerich JE, Bolli GB. Comparison of glucose counterregulation during short-term and prolonged hypoglycemia in normal humans. *Diabetes* 1986;35:563–569

113. Cryer PE. Glucose counterregulation in man. *Diabetes* 1981;30:261–264

114. Gerich JE. Glucose counterregulation and its impact on diabetes mellitus. *Diabetes* 1988;37:1608–1617

115. De Feo P, Perriello G, Torlone E, Fanelli C, Ventura MM, Santeusanio F, Brunetti P, Gerich JE, Bolli GB. Evidence against important catecholamine compensation for absent glucagon counterregulation. *Am J Physiol Endocrinol Metab* 1991;260:E203–E212

116. De Feo P, Perriello G, Torlone E, Fanelli C, Ventura MM, Santeusanio F, Brunetti P, Gerich JE, Bolli GB. Contribution of adrenergic mechanisms to glucose counterregulation in humans. *Am J Physiol Endocrinol Metab* 1991;261:E725–E736

117. Rosen SG, Clutter WE, Berk MA, Shah SD, Cryer PE. Epinephrine supports the postabsorptive plasma glucose concentration and prevents hypoglycemia when glucagon secretion is deficient in man. *J Clin Invest* 1984;73:405–411

118. Boyle PJ, Shah SD, Cryer PE. Insulin, glucagon, and catecholamines in prevention of hypoglycemia during fasting in humans. *Am J Physiol Endocrinol Metab* 1989;256:E651–E661

119. Tse TF, Clutter WE, Shah SD, Cryer PE. Mechanisms of postprandial glucose counterregulation in man: physiologic roles of glucagon and epinephrine vis-à-vis insulin in the prevention of hypoglycemia late after glucose ingestion. *J Clin Invest* 1983;72:278–286

120. Tse TF, Clutter WE, Shah SD, Miller JP, Cryer PE. Neuroendocrine responses to glucose ingestion in man: specificity, temporal relationships and quantitative aspects. *J Clin Invest* 1983;72:270–277

121. Hirsch IB, Marker JC, Smith L, Spina RJ, Parvin CA, Holloszy JO, Cryer PE. Insulin and glucagon in the prevention of hypoglycemia during exercise in humans. *Am J Physiol Endocrinol Metab* 1991;260:E695–E704

122. Marker JC, Hirsch IB, Smith L, Parvin CA, Holloszy JO, Cryer PE. Catecholamines in the prevention of hypoglycemia during exercise in humans. *Am J Physiol Endocrinol Metab* 1991;260:E705–E712

123. De Feo P, Perriello G, Torlone E, Ventura MM, Santeusanio F, Brunetti P, Gerich JE, Bolli GB. Demonstration of a role for growth hormone in glucose counterregulation. *Am J Physiol Endocrinol Metab* 1989;256:E835–E843

124. De Feo P, Perriello G, Torlone E, Ventura MM, Fanelli C, Santeusanio F, Brunetti P, Gerich JE, Bolli GB. Contribution of cortisol to glucose counterregulation in humans. *Am J Physiol Endocrinol Metab* 1989;257:E35–E42

125. Boyle PJ, Cryer PE. Growth hormone, cortisol, or both are involved in defense against, but are not critical to recovery from, hypoglycemia. *Am J Physiol Endocrinol Metab* 1991;260:E395–E402

126. Bolli G, De Feo P, Perriello G, De Cosmo S, Ventura M, Campbell P, Brunetti P, Gerich JE. Role of hepatic autoregulation in defense against hypoglycemia in humans. *J Clin Invest* 1985;75:162–163

127. Fanelli CG, De Feo P, Porcellati F, Perriello G, Torlone E, Santeusanio F, Brunetti P, Bolli GB. Adrenergic mechanisms contribute to the late phase of hypoglycemic glucose counterregulation in humans by stimulating lipolysis. *J Clin Invest* 1992;89:2005–2013

128. Cryer PE. Mechanisms of sympathoadrenal failure and hypoglycemia in diabetes. *J Clin Invest* 2006;116:1470–1473

129. Watts AG, Donovan CM. Sweet talk in the brain: glucosensing neural networks, and hypoglycemic counterregulation. *Front Neuroendocrinol* 2010;31:32-43

130. Teves D, Videen TO, Cryer PE, Powers WJ. Activation of human medial prefrontal cortex during autonomic responses to hypoglycemia. *Proc Natl Acad Sci USA* 2004;101:6217–6221

131. Arbeláez AM, Powers WJ, Videen TO, Price JL, Cryer PE. Attenuation of counterregulatory responses to recurrent hypoglycemia by active thalamic inhibition. A mechanism for hypoglycemia-associated autonomic failure. *Diabetes* 2008;57:470–475

132. Arbeláez AM, Rutlin JR, Hershey Y, Powers WJ, Videen TO, Cryer PE. Thalamic activation during slightly subphysiological glycemia in humans. *Diabetes Care* 2012;35:2570–2574

133. Chan O, Sherwin R. Influence of VMH fuel sensing on hypoglycemic responses. *Trends Endocrinol Metab* 2013;24:616–624

3
The Pathophysiology of Glucose Counterregulation in Diabetes

Overview: Interplay of Insulin Excess and Compromised Glucose Counterregulation

As developed in Chapter 1, iatrogenic hypoglycemia is the limiting factor in the glycemic management of diabetes. It causes recurrent morbidity in most people with type 1 diabetes (T1D) and many with advanced (absolute endogenous insulin–deficient) type 2 diabetes (T2D), and it is sometimes fatal. In addition, it generally precludes maintenance of euglycemia over a lifetime of diabetes and thus full realization of the vascular benefits of long-term glycemic control. Furthermore, as discussed in this chapter, it compromises defenses against subsequent hypoglycemia and thus causes a vicious cycle of recurrent hypoglycemia.

Hypoglycemia in diabetes is typically the result of the interplay of relative or absolute therapeutic insulin excess and compromised defenses against falling plasma glucose concentrations.[1–6] Thus, it is fundamentally iatrogenic, the result of treatments that raise circulating insulin levels and thus lower plasma glucose concentrations (see Chapter 2). Those treatments include insulin and insulin secretagogues such as a sulfonylurea (e.g., glyburide [glibenclamide], glipizide, glimepiride, or gliclazide, among others) or a glinide (e.g., nateglinide, repaglinide). All people with T1D must be treated with insulin.

DOI: 10.2337/9781580406499.03

Many people with T2D ultimately require treatment with insulin.[7] Early in the course of the disease, individuals with T2D may respond to treatment with an insulin secretagogue. Alternatively, they may respond to drugs that do not raise insulin levels, at least when plasma glucose concentrations fall into and below the physiological range. The latter include a biguanide (metformin), thiazolidinediones (e.g., pioglitazone, rosiglitazone), α-glucosidase inhibitors (e.g., acarbose, miglitol), glucagon-like peptide-1 receptor agonists (e.g., exenatide, liraglutide, albiglitude, lixisenatide, dulaglutide), dipeptidyl peptidase-IV inhibitors (e.g., sitagliptin, saxagliptin, vildagliptin, linagliptin, alogliptin), and sodium-glucose cotransporter 2 (SGLT2) inhibitors (e.g., canagliflozin, dapagliflozin, empagliflozin, and others). These drugs should not, and probably do not,[8–11] cause hypoglycemia when used as monotherapy, although metformin has been reported to cause self-reported hypoglycemia,[12,13] or when used in combination among themselves (see Chapter 1). These drugs, however, can increase the risk of hypoglycemia when used with insulin or with a sulfonylurea.

Insulin Excess

Relative or even absolute insulin excess must occur from time to time during treatment with an insulin secretagogue or with insulin because of the pharmacokinetic imperfections of these therapies. Even the most sophisticated regimens do not replicate normal (endogenous) insulin secretion, which is plasma glucose–regulated and during which variations in circulating insulin levels occur over minutes. With an insulin secretagogue or insulin, to the extent the patient has deficient endogenous insulin secretion, insulin levels are not plasma-glucose regulated. Furthermore, variations in insulin levels occur over hours.

Insulin excess of sufficient magnitude can cause hypoglycemia. As developed in Chapter 1, the frequency of hypoglycemia is relatively low (at least with currently recommended glycemic goals) even during therapy with insulin early in the course of T2D.[14] (Indeed, it is relatively low early in the course of T1D—the "honeymoon" period.) Therefore, factors in addition to relative or absolute therapeutic insulin excess must play an important role in the pathogenesis of hypoglycemia, which becomes progressively more frequent over time—rapidly in T1D and gradually in T2D (see Chapter 1). Those additional factors are progressive failure of the normal physiological and behavioral defenses against falling plasma glucose concentrations (see Chapter 2). Thus, although therapeutic hyperinsulinemia—either relative (to low rates of exogenous or endogenous glucose flux into the circulation or high rates of glucose flux out of the circulation) or absolute—is a prerequisite for the development of hypoglycemia in diabetes, compromised glucose counterregulation is the key feature of the pathogenesis of iatrogenic hypoglycemia in T1D and advanced T2D. Hypoglycemia in diabetes is typically the result of the interplay of relative or absolute therapeutic insulin excess and compromised physiological and behavioral defenses against falling plasma glucose concentrations.[1–3,5,6]

Compromised Glucose Counterregulation

As discussed in Chapter 2, the key physiological defenses against falling plasma glucose concentrations (Figure 2.5) are as follows: *1*) decrements in pancreatic islet β-cell insulin secretion; *2*) increments in pancreatic islet α-cell glucagon secretion, and, absent the latter; *3*) increments in adrenomedullary epinephrine secretion.[2,3,5,6,15] The behavioral defense is the ingestion of carbohydrates prompted by symptoms—largely neurogenic symptoms[16]—that make the individual aware of hypoglycemia.[2,3,5,6,15] All of these defenses are typically compromised in T1D and advanced T2D.[1,2,3,5,6,17,18]

In fully developed (i.e., absolutely or nearly C-peptide–negative) T1D, circulating insulin levels do not decrease as plasma glucose concentrations decline through or below the physiological range. In the absence of functioning β-cells, plasma insulin levels are simply a passive function of the clearance of administered (exogenous) insulin. Furthermore, in the absence of a β-cell signal, that is, a decrease in intraislet insulin perhaps among other β-cell secretory products,[3,19–25] circulating glucagon levels do not increase as plasma glucose concentrations fall below the physiological range (Figure 3.1).[26] Thus, both the first defense against hypoglycemia—a decrease in insulin levels—and the second defense against hypoglycemia—an increase in glucagon levels—are lost in T1D. Therefore, patients with T1D are critically dependent on the third defense against hypoglycemia, an increase in epinephrine levels. The epinephrine secretory response to hypoglycemia, however, typically is attenuated in T1D (Figure 3.1).[1–3,5,6,17,27] Through mechanisms yet to be clearly defined but often thought to reside in the brain,[1–3,5,6,28,29] the glycemic threshold for sympathoadrenal—both adrenomedullary and sympathetic neural—activation is

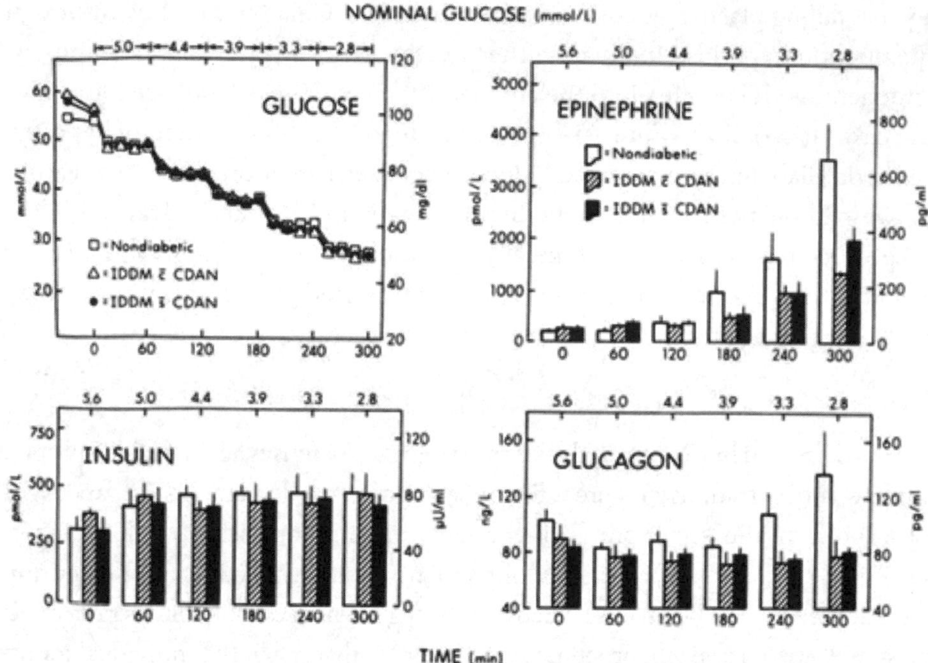

Figure 3.1—Mean (±SE) plasma glucose, insulin, epinephrine, and glucagon concentrations during hyperinsulinemic stepped hypoglycemia glucose clamps in individuals without diabetes (open squares and columns), people with type 1 diabetes with classical diabetic autonomic neuropathy (CDAN; open triangles and cross-hatched columns), and people with type 1 diabetes without CDAN (closed circles and columns).

Source: From Dagogo-Jack et al.[17] with permission from the American Society for Clinical Investigation.

shifted to lower plasma glucose concentrations by recent antecedent hypoglycemia (Figures 3.2 and 3.3),[17,18,30] as well as by prior exercise[31–33] and by sleep.[34–36]

The patterns of plasma insulin, glucagon, and epinephrine responses to falling plasma glucose concentrations in nondiabetic individuals, people with T1D, and T2D are summarized in Table 3.1. The reduced responses to a given level of hypoglycemia cause the clinical syndromes of defective glucose counterregulation and hypoglycemia unawareness.[1–3,5,6]

Table 3.1—Responses to Falling Plasma Glucose Concentrations in Humans

Plasma glucose	Individuals	Plasma		
	—	Insulin	Glucagon	Epinephrine
↓	Without diabetes	↓	↑	↑
↓	Type 1 diabetes	No ↓	No ↑	Attenuated ↑
• Defective glucose counterregulation • Hypoglycemia unawareness				
↓	Type 2 diabetes – Early	↓	↑	↑
↓	Type 2 diabetes – Late	No ↓	No ↑	Attenuated ↑

Defective Glucose Counterregulation

In the setting of absent decrements in insulin and absent increments in glucagon, attenuated increments in epinephrine as plasma glucose levels fall in response to therapeutic hyperinsulinemia cause the clinical syndrome of defective glucose counterregulation (Table 3.1).[1–3,5,6] Compared with patients with T1D who have absent insulin and glucagon responses but normal epinephrine responses, patients with absent insulin and glucagon responses and reduced epinephrine responses have been shown to be at 25-fold[37] or greater[38] increased risk for severe iatrogenic hypoglycemia during aggressive glycemic therapy. Originally identified by the failure of glycemic defense against low-dose insulin infusions,[37,38] the clinical syndrome of defective glucose counterregulation is characterized by absent decrements in insulin, absent increments in glucagon, and attenuated increments in epinephrine at a given level of hypoglycemia in insulin-deficient diabetes (Figure 3.1).[1–3,5,6,17]

Hypoglycemia Unawareness

An attenuated epinephrine response to hypoglycemia (see Table 3.1 and Figure 3.1) is a marker of an attenuated sympathoadrenal—sympathetic neural as well as adrenomedullary—response. Largely as a result of an attenuated sympathetic neural response,[16] the attenuated sympathoadrenal response causes the clinical syndrome of hypoglycemia unawareness— impairment or even complete loss of the warning, largely neurogenic symptoms that previously prompted the behavioral defense (i.e., the ingestion of carbohydrates). Hypoglycemia unawareness—or more precisely impaired awareness of hypoglycemia—is common in T1D and is associated with low plasma glucose concentrations whether those are assessed by A1C levels[39] or by continuous glucose monitoring.[40] It is associated with a sixfold or greater increased risk for severe hypoglycemia.[41,42] In one study, patients with T1D and impaired awareness of hypoglycemia were found to suffer many more episodes of asymptomatic hypoglycemia than those with intact awareness and were tenfold more likely (53% vs. 5%) to suffer severe hypoglycemia.[43] The estimated incidence of severe hypoglycemia was increased from 1.0 per patient-year in aware individuals to 16.0 per patient-year in those with impaired awareness of hypoglycemia.

It is generally thought that hypoglycemia unawareness is due to reduced release of the sympathetic neural neurotransmitters norepinephrine and acetylcholine and perhaps also that of adrenomedullary epinephrine.[16] This belief is consistent with the findings that electroencephalogram (EEG) changes and cognitive dysfunction and higher brain functions during hypoglycemia are not different in patients with and without hypoglycemia unawareness.[44] However, there is evidence of decreased β-adrenergic sensitivity—specifically, reduced cardiac chronotropic sensitivity to isoproterenol[45,46]—in patients with unawareness. But vascular sensitivity to infusion of a β_2-adrenergic agonist was not found to be reduced in patients with unawareness[47] or following recent antecedent hypoglycemia in individuals without diabetes.[48] Furthermore, reduced symptomatic β-adrenergic sensitivity remains to be demonstrated specifically in patients with such unawareness. Finally, it also would be necessary to postulate reduced cholinergic sensitivity to explain reduced cholinergic symptoms, such as sweating.

Hypoglycemia-Associated Autonomic Failure

On the basis of the pivotal finding that a 2-h episode of afternoon hyperinsulinemic hypoglycemia, compared with afternoon hyperinsulinemic euglycemia, reduced the sympathoadrenal and symptomatic (among other) responses to hypoglycemia the following morning in individuals without diabetes,[30] the concept of hypoglycemia-associated autonomic failure (HAAF) in diabetes[1–3,5,6,17,18,31–36] was formulated[49] and then documented in patients with T1D[17] and advanced T2D.[18] The effects of prior hypoglycemia on the responses to subsequent hypoglycemia in patients with T1D are illustrated in Figures 3.2 and 3.3.

The concept of HAAF in diabetes[1–3,5,6] posits that recent antecedent hypoglycemia,[17,18,28,50] as well as prior exercise[31–33] and sleep,[34–36] cause both defective glucose counterregulation (by reducing the adrenomedullary epinephrine

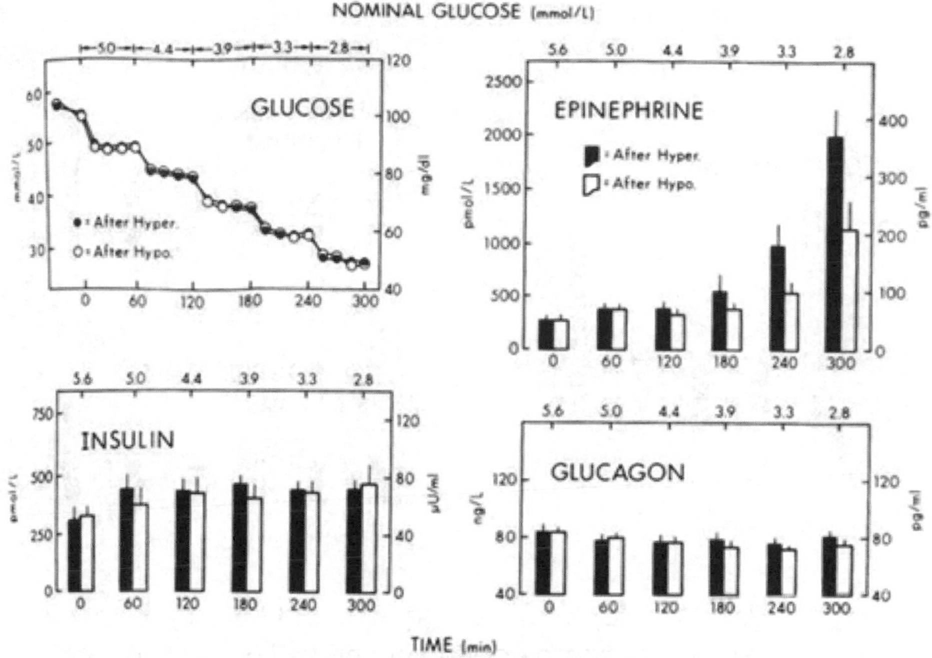

Figure 3.2—Mean (+SE) plasma glucose, insulin, epinephrine, and glucagon concentrations during hyperinsulinemic stepped hypoglycemic glucose clamps in patients with type 1 diabetes (IDD, insulin-dependent diabetes) without classical diabetic autonomic neuropathy on mornings following afternoon hyperglycemia (After Hyper., closed circles and columns) and on mornings following afternoon hypoglycemia (After Hypo., open circles and columns).

Source: From Dagogo-Jack et al.[17] with permission from the American Society for Clinical Investigation.

response in the absence of decrements in insulin and increments in glucagon; see Figure 3.2) and hypoglycemia unawareness (by reducing the sympathoadrenal, including the sympathetic neural, and the resulting neurogenic symptom responses; see Figure 3.3) and therefore a vicious cycle of recurrent hypoglycemia. The concept of HAAF is illustrated in Figure 3.4.

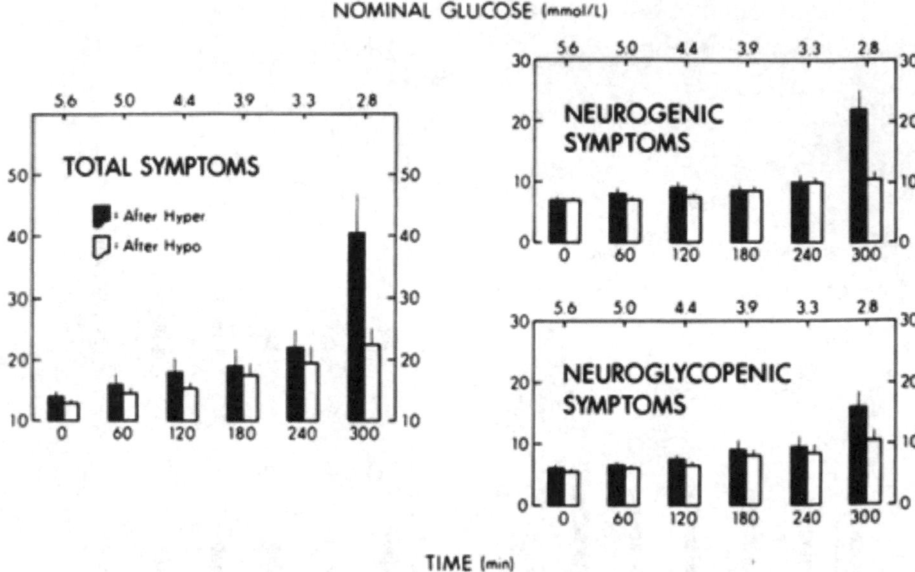

Figure 3.3—Mean (+SE) total, neurogenic, and neuroglycopenic symptom scores during hyperinsulinemic stepped hypoglycemic clamps in patients with type 1 diabetes (IDD, insulin-dependent diabetes) without classical diabetic autonomic neuropathy on mornings following afternoon hyperglycemia (After hyper., closed columns) and on mornings following afternoon hypoglycemia (After hypo., open columns).

Source: From Dagogo-Jack et al.[17] with permission from the American Society for Clinical Investigation.

Absolute therapeutic insulin excess of sufficient magnitude can cause an isolated episode of hypoglycemia even in early T2D with relative insulin deficiency and, therefore, intact insulin and glucagon responses to falling plasma glucose concentrations (Figure 3.4). Hypoglycemia is infrequent in such individuals. Conversely, mild to moderate or even relative (to a low rate of glucose influx into the circulation, a high rate of glucose efflux out of the circulation, or both) therapeutic insulin excess often causes hypoglycemia in individuals with absolute endogenous insulin deficiency—advanced T2D or T1D—and the resulting loss of insulin and glucagon responses to falling plasma glucose levels. In

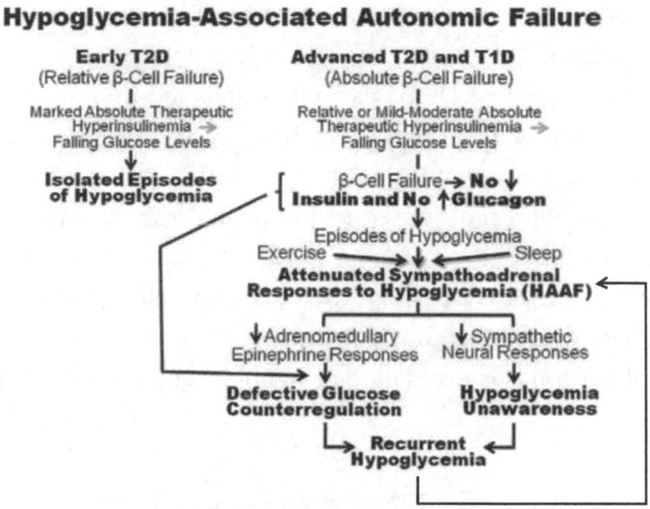

Figure 3.4—Schematic diagram of hypoglycemia-associated autonomic failure (HAAF) in diabetes.

Source: Modified from Cryer.[1]

the latter setting, episodes of recent antecedent hypoglycemia, or sleep or prior exercise, result in the addition of an attenuated sympathoadrenal response to falling plasma glucose levels and, thus, produce the clinical syndromes of defective glucose counterregulation and hypoglycemia unawareness (Figure 3.4) and recurrent iatrogenic hypoglycemia.

HAAF is a functional disorder distinct from classical diabetic autonomic neuropathy.[17,51] It is a dynamic phenomenon that can be induced (by prior hypoglycemia or exercise or sleep) and largely reversed (by avoidance of hypoglycemia) and is manifested clinically by recurrent iatrogenic hypoglycemia. In contrast, diabetic autonomic neuropathy is a structural disorder that is manifested clinically by gastrointestinal or genitourinary symptoms, by orthostatic hypotension, or by combinations of these and is not reversible. Nonetheless, evidence has shown that the key feature of HAAF—an attenuated sympathoadrenal response to a given level of hypoglycemia—is more prominent in patients with diabetic autonomic neuropathy.[52,53] That is illustrated in Figure 3.1.[17] Indeed, recent antecedent hypoglycemia reduces sympathoadrenal responses to subsequent hemodynamic stimuli and also reduces baroreflex sensitivity.[54,55] Thus, HAAF includes a form of autonomic failure functionally analogous to autonomic neuropathy with respect to cardiovascular, as well as metabolic, regulation.

The clinical impact of HAAF is well established in T1D.[17,37,38,41,56–61] For example, recent antecedent hypoglycemia, even asymptomatic nocturnal hypoglycemia, reduces epinephrine, symptomatic, and cognitive dysfunction responses to a given level of subsequent hypoglycemia[59]; reduces detection of hypoglycemia in the clinical setting[60]; and reduces glycemic defense against hyperinsulinemia[17] in T1D. Perhaps the most compelling support for the concept of HAAF is the finding, in three independent laboratories, that as few as 2–3 weeks of scrupulous avoidance of hypoglycemia reverses hypoglycemia

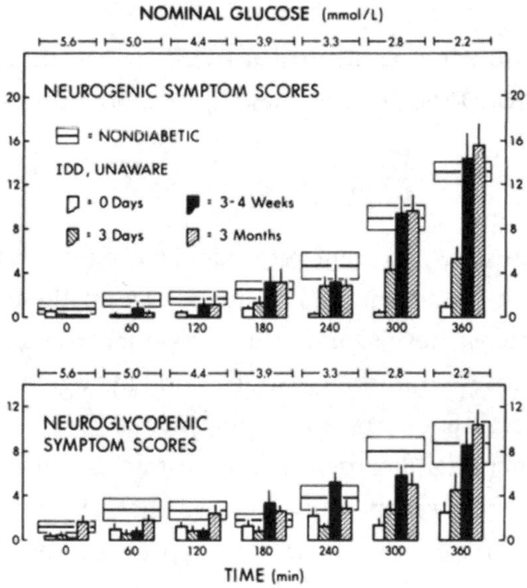

Figure 3.5—Mean (+SE) neurogenic and neuroglycopenic symptom scores during hyperinsulinemic stepped hypoglycemic clamps in individuals without diabetes (rectangles) and in patients with type 1 diabetes (IDD, insulin-dependent diabetes) (columns) at baseline (0 days), after 3 days of inpatient strict avoidance of hypoglycemia, and after 3–4 weeks and 3 months of outpatient scrupulous avoidance of hypoglycemia.

Source: Dagogo-Jack et al.[56] with permission from the American Diabetes Association.

unawareness (see Figure 3.5) and improves the reduced epinephrine component of defective glucose counterregulation in most affected patients.[56–58,61] In addition, successful islet transplantation in T1D—which eliminates or reduces a need for therapy with exogenous insulin and thus eliminates or reduces iatrogenic hypoglycemia—partially restores decrements in insulin and increments in glucagon and epinephrine, symptoms, and endogenous glucose production during hypoglycemia.[62,63]

Developed initially in T1D,[17] the concept of HAAF has been extended to T2D.[18] In advanced (i.e., absolute endogenous insulin–deficient) T2D, glucagon responses to hypoglycemia are lost,[18] as they are in T1D. Furthermore, the glycemic thresholds for epinephrine and symptom responses (among other responses) are shifted to lower plasma glucose concentrations by recent antecedent hypoglycemia in T2D,[18,64] as they are in T1D. Thus, people with advanced T2D are also at risk for HAAF.

The findings that people with relatively mild T2D reasonably but not fully controlled with diet or oral antidiabetic agents have estimated glycemic thresholds for glucose counterregulatory hormone[65,66] and symptomatic[65,67] responses to hypoglycemia at higher plasma glucose concentrations than individuals without diabetes are likely the result of the pathophysiology of glucose counterregulation in diabetes rather than a unique feature of T2D. These findings are plausibly attributed to the fact that these individuals with T2D have higher mean plasma glucose concentrations, which raise the glycemic thresholds to higher plasma glucose levels (and have fewer episodes of iatrogenic hypoglycemia that would shift the glycemic thresholds to lower plasma glucose levels),[68,69] as discussed earlier.

The pathophysiology of glucose counterregulation, and thus the pathogenesis of iatrogenic hypoglycemia, is basically the same in T1D and T2D. Iatrogenic hypoglycemia is typically the result of the interplay of therapeutic hyperinsulinemia and compromised defenses against falling plasma glucose concentrations (HAAF in diabetes). Because HAAF stems fundamentally from β-cell failure,[2,3,5,6,20,24] which results in loss of both the insulin and glucagon responses, setting the stage for the effect of attenuated sympathoadrenal responses to cause defective glucose counterregulation, as well as hypoglycemia unawareness, it develops rapidly in T1D (in which β-cell failure develops rapidly) but slowly in T2D (in which absolute β-cell failure develops slowly). This result explains the relatively low frequency of hypoglycemia (at least with currently recommended glycemic goals) early in the course of T2D and the relatively high frequency of hypoglycemia, approaching that in T1D, as patients approach the insulin-deficient end of the spectrum of T2D (see Chapter 1).

Diverse Causes of HAAF

Diverse causes of HAAF in diabetes are now recognized (Figure 3.4).[1–3,5,6] Those causes include *1*) HAAF induced by recent antecedent iatrogenic hypoglycemia—hypoglycemia-related HAAF,[17,18] 2) HAAF induced by prior exercise—exercise-related HAAF,[31–33] and 3) HAAF induced by sleep—sleep-related HAAF.[34–36] Each of these inciting events causes reduced sympathoadrenal and symptomatic responses to a given level of subsequent hypoglycemia, which is the key feature of HAAF (i.e., sympathoadrenal failure associated with the development of iatrogenic hypoglycemia in diabetes). Indeed, it is conceivable that additional causes of HAAF exist.

Hypoglycemia-Related HAAF

As discussed in this chapter, recent antecedent iatrogenic hypoglycemia was the first recognized cause of HAAF and led to the concept (see Figure 3.5).[1–3,5,6,17,18]

Exercise-Related HAAF

Exercise increases glucose utilization (by exercising muscle). In nondiabetic individuals, decrements in insulin, increments in glucagon, and increments in catecholamines (during intense exercise) result in increases in glucose production that generally match or even exceed those in glucose utilization, and hypoglycemia does not occur.[33] Largely because insulin levels are unregulated, hypoglycemia occurs commonly during or shortly after exercise in people with T1D.[70] Interestingly, the risk of hypoglycemia appears to be higher during late afternoon, compared with prebreakfast, exercise.[71]

The risk of hypoglycemia during or shortly after exercise in T1D generally is recognized, but the risk of late postexercise hypoglycemia is less widely appreciated.[72,73] Postexercise late-onset hypoglycemia in patients with T1D, typically nocturnal and occurring 6–15 h after unusually strenuous exercise, was nicely described by MacDonald[72] nearly three decades ago. In one study, a quarter of patients with T1D suffered nocturnal hypoglycemia in the absence of exercise the previous afternoon, and half of the patients suffered nocturnal hypoglycemia after exercise the previous afternoon.[73] It has been estimated that an adolescent with T1D who accumulated the recommended 60 min/day of moderate to vigorous physical activity would have a 104 and a 72% higher risk of hypoglycemia overnight and the following day, respectively, compared with no such activity.[74] These findings follow directly from the pathophysiology of glucose counterregulation.[31–33] Younk and Davis[75] have reported that exercise reduces sympathoadrenal responses to a given level of hypoglycemia several hours later in both nondiabetic individuals[31] and people with T1D.[32] The latter's insulin and glucagon responses are absent and their sympathoadrenal and symptomatic responses to hypoglycemia are reduced; additionally, their sympathoadrenal responses are reduced further after exercise.[32] They have exercise-related HAAF[33] and, therefore, an increased risk of hypoglycemia.[73]

Sleep-Related HAAF

In people with T1D, sympathoadrenal responses to a given level of hypoglycemia are reduced further during sleep.[34,35] Perhaps because of their further reduced sympathoadrenal responses, they are much less likely to be awakened by hypoglycemia than nondiabetic individuals.[35,36] Thus, sleeping patients with T1D have both further reduced epinephrine responses to hypoglycemia, the key feature of defective glucose counterregulation, and reduced arousal from sleep, a form of hypoglycemia unawareness. They have sleep-related HAAF[34–36] and are at high risk for hypoglycemia.[76] Reduced awakening during nocturnal hypoglycemia has also been reported in T2D.[77]

Additional Causes of HAAF

There may be as yet unrecognized functional, and thus potentially reversible, causes of HAAF in addition to recent antecedent hypoglycemia, prior exercise, and sleep. Furthermore, there may well be a structural factor, because the adrenal medullae can be conceptualized as postganglionic neurons without axons and therefore could be subject to neuropathy.[17,52,53] Indeed, there are clues to a fixed reduction of the epinephrine response to a given level of hypoglycemia in people with longstanding T1D. First, although it reverses hypoglycemia unawareness, scrupulous avoidance of iatrogenic hypoglycemia improves but does not fully normalize the plasma epinephrine response to hypoglycemia.[56–58,61] Second, when it is successful by producing insulin independence, islet transplantation virtually eliminates hypoglycemia and normalizes the glycemic threshold for epinephrine secretion and increases its magnitude, but it does not appear to fully normalize the magnitude of the epinephrine response.[62,63] Third, as mentioned earlier, the epinephrine response to hypoglycemia is reduced to a greater extent in patients with clinically apparent classical diabetic autonomic neuropathy than it is in individuals without overt evidence of that complication.[52,53] Indeed, the frequency of severe hypoglycemia is increased in patients with classical diabetic autonomic neuropathy.[78] Fourth, the finding of a reduced plasma metanephrine, as well as epinephrine, response to hypoglycemia in patients with HAAF suggests a reduced adrenomedullary epinephrine secretory capacity.[79]

Mechanisms of HAAF

HAAF develops in the setting of absent decrements in insulin and absent increments in glucagon as plasma glucose concentrations fall in response to therapeutic hyperinsulinemia in T1D and advanced T2D.[1–3,5,6] The mechanisms of these prerequisite abnormalities are different from those of the attenuated sympathoadrenal and resulting symptomatic responses to hypoglycemia that ultimately cause the clinical syndromes of defective glucose counterregulation and hypoglycemia unawareness, the components of HAAF,

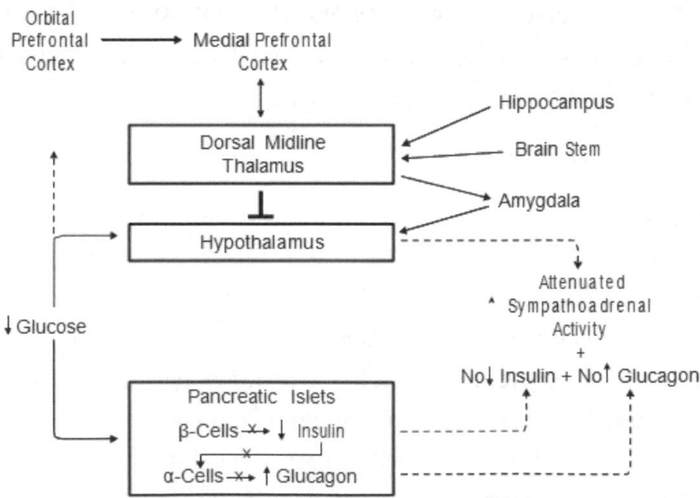

Figure 3.6—Pancreatic islet, hypothalamic, and cerebral network mechanisms of hypoglycemic-associated autonomic failure (HAAF) in diabetes. Compare with Figure 2.6.

as discussed earlier. These mechanisms are summarized in Figure 3.6 and have been discussed in detail.[3]

Absent Insulin and Glucagon Responses

The glucagon response to hypoglycemia is lost in T1D.[26] It is lost early, before the sympathoadrenal response becomes attenuated[27]; indeed, it is attenuated within the first year of T1D.[80] Its loss is independent of diabetic autonomic neuropathy[17] (see Figure 3.1) and is not corrected by scrupulous avoidance of hypoglycemia.[56–58,61]

Because both T1D and advanced (i.e., absolute endogenous insulin deficient) T2D are the result of pancreatic islet β-cell failure, the mechanism of the loss of a decrement in insulin as plasma glucose concentrations decline within and below the physiological range is straightforward.[3] In the absence of endogenous insulin secretion, circulating insulin concentrations are simply the result of the absorption and clearance of injected insulin. Insulin levels are not glucose regulated and do not decrease as glucose levels fall. The mechanism of the loss of the increment in glucagon is less clear-cut.[3]

The absence of an increase in α-cell glucagon secretion in response to hypoglycemia in absolute endogenous insulin deficiency is also best attributed to β-cell failure, specifically the absence of a decrease in the α-cell inhibitory signal of β-cell insulin. The evidence for that conclusion has been reviewed and summarized.[3,25]

Glucagon secretory responses to administered amino acids occur in patients with insulin-deficient diabetes who have no glucagon response to hypoglycemia.[81–84] Therefore, loss of the glucagon response to falling plasma glucose concentrations in T1D[17,26,27,37,56,57,59,60,85] and advanced T2D[18] must be the result of a defect in signaling to functional glucagon-secreting pancreatic islet α-cells. (The extent to which the reduced absolute glucagon response to administered amino acids in T1D[81,82,84] is the result of reduced glucagon secretion per α-cell, a reduced α-cell mass, or both is unknown.)

As discussed in Chapter 2, the normal regulation of α-cell glucagon secretion is complex and incompletely understood (e.g., see Cooperberg and Cryer[23,24]). Evidence is now substantial that β-cell secretory products normally inhibit α-cell glucagon secretion and that a decrease in β-cell secretion, including a decrease in insulin secretion, signals an increase in α-cell glucagon secretion during hypoglycemia in humans.[19–24] Thus, it follows that β-cell failure causes loss of the glucagon secretory response to hypoglycemia early in T1D and later in T2D (Figure 3.6).[1–3,5,6] That construct is supported by the findings that *1*) the degree of loss of glucagon secretion is associated with the degree of loss of insulin secretion,[85] *2*) an increase in glucagon secretion can be triggered by a decrease in (exogenous) insulin during hypoglycemia in T1D,[24] and *3*) the normal inverse relationship between pulses of insulin and glucagon secretion is lost in T2D.[86]

Loss of the glucagon response to hypoglycemia in absolute endogenous insulin–deficient diabetes cannot be attributed to loss of islet nerves[87] or to loss of central nervous system (CNS)–derived neural signaling.[88] Quantitatively normal glucagon secretory responses to hypoglycemia occur from the denervated (transplanted) human pancreas[89] and from the denervated dog pancreas[90] as well as in patients with spinal cord transections and, therefore, no sympathoadrenal outflow to the islets.[91] Qualitatively normal glucagon secretory responses to low glucose levels occur from the perfused rodent pancreas[92] and from perifused rodent and human islets.[93] Furthermore, adrenergic blockade does not prevent the glucagon response to hypoglycemia in humans[94] and epinephrine-deficient bilaterally adrenalectomized individuals have a normal glucagon response to hypoglycemia.[16] The role of glucagon in the pathogenesis of hypoglycemia (and hyperglycemia) in diabetes has been reviewed.[25]

An intraislet mechanism other than β-cell failure could be inhibition of glucagon secretion by excessive δ-cell somatostatin release during hypoglycemia in diabetes. It has been reported that infusion of a somatostatin receptor-2 antagonist increased the glucagon secretory response to hypoglycemia in streptozotocin diabetic rats.[95,96] The antagonist, however, did not consistently decrease the glucose infusion rate required to maintain the hypoglycemic clamps, raised glucagon levels during euglycemia, and paradoxically decreased the glucagon response to hypoglycemia in nondiabetic rats. In a subsequent study in biobreeding diabetic rats,[97] the somatostatin antagonist decreased the required glucose infusion rates during hypoglycemia, but it increased the glucagon secretory response to hypoglycemia to a similar extent in nondiabetic and diabetic animals, and it increased glucagon release from pancreatic slices obtained from nondiabetic and diabetic rats at normal as well as low glucose concentrations and in response to arginine. Thus, although the data confirm that somatostatin inhibits glucagon secretion, they are not consistent with the notion that a specific defect results in excessive intraislet somatostatin release during hypoglycemia that is unique to diabetes and therefore explains the selective loss of the glucagon response to hypoglycemia in diabetes.

These data support the conclusion that in absolute endogenous insulin–deficient diabetes (T1D or advanced T2D), the absence of a decrease in β-cell insulin secretion causes a loss of an increase in α-cell glucagon secretion as glucose concentrations fall in response to therapeutic hyperinsulinemia. The absence of a decrease in insulin and of an increase in glucagon are prerequisite to defective glucose counterregulation, but they do not cause defective glucose counterregulation or hypoglycemia unawareness. Those two components of HAAF in diabetes develop only when the sympathoadrenal and symptomatic responses to hypoglycemia become attenuated (Figures 3.4 and 3.6).[3]

Attenuated Sympathoadrenal Responses

The mechanisms of the key component of HAAF in diabetes, the attenuated CNS-mediated sympathoadrenal response to falling plasma glucose concentrations, is not known. The attenuated sympathoadrenal response causes hypoglycemia unawareness and, in the setting of absent decrements in insulin and absent increments in glucagon, the attenuated adrenomedullary epinephrine response causes defective glucose counterregulation, and thus HAAF and iatrogenic hypoglycemia in T1D and advanced T2D.[1–3,5,6,17,18] Clearly, however, the mechanism is different from that of loss of the insulin and glucagon responses to hypoglycemia, because the latter responses occur primarily at the level of the diseased pancreatic islets, whereas the attenuated sympathoadrenal response involves the CNS (Figure 3.6).

Theoretically, the alteration that causes the glycemic thresholds for the sympathoadrenal and symptomatic (among other) responses to shift to lower plasma glucose concentrations after recent antecedent hypoglycemia (or after exercise and during sleep) could be in the CNS or in the afferent or efferent components of the sympathoadrenal system. Indeed, the finding of a reduced plasma metanephrine response to hypoglycemia in patients with T1D and HAAF suggests a reduced adrenomedullary capacity to secrete epinephrine.[79] HAAF is mediated through adrenergic mechanisms.[98] Combined α- and β-adrenergic blockade prevents the effect of hypoglycemia to attenuate the sympathoadrenal response to subsequent hypoglycemia. Interestingly, evidence indicates that ventromedial hypothalamic β_2-adrenergic stimulation increases the plasma epinephrine response to hypoglycemia in rats.[99]

Potential CNS mechanisms include *1*) the systemic mediator hypothesis, *2*) the brain fuel transport hypothesis, *3*) the brain metabolism hypothesis, and *4*) the cerebral network hypothesis.[3,100–102] Most of the postulated mechanisms of HAAF are based on sophisticated studies in rodents. Barriers to the study of the mechanisms of HAAF in humans include *1*) limited methods to measure human brain function noninvasively and *2*) the failure of investigators to clearly define patients with HAAF and patients without HAAF and to include nondiabetic controls.[3] The former problem is beginning to yield to positron emission tomography (PET) and magnetic resonance imaging and spectroscopy.

The *systemic mediator hypothesis* posits that increased circulating cortisol levels (or perhaps those of another systemic factor) during recent antecedent hypoglycemia (or exercise) act on the brain to reduce the sympathoadrenal (among other) responses to a given level of subsequent hypoglycemia.[3] Substantial antecedent cortisol elevations, produced by cortisol infusion or ACTH administration, do reduce the sympathoadrenal and symptomatic responses to subsequent hypoglycemia.[103–105] That appears to be an effect of supraphysiological cortisol concentrations. Less marked plasma cortisol elevations, to levels comparable to those that occur during hypoglycemia, do not reduce adrenomedullary or symptomatic responses to subsequent hypoglycemia.[106,107] Furthermore, inhibition of the cortisol response to antecedent hypoglycemia (with metyrapone) does not prevent the effect of antecedent hypoglycemia to reduce the sympathoadrenal (or other) responses to subsequent hypoglycemia.[107] Cortisol infusions leading to plasma cortisol concentrations similar to those that occur during hypoglycemia have been reported to blunt sympathoadrenal (among other) responses to subsequent exercise.[108] Evidence also indicates that antecedent plasma epinephrine elevations do not cause HAAF.[109]

The *brain fuel transport hypothesis* posits that recent antecedent hypoglycemia causes increased blood-to-brain transport of glucose (or of an alternative metabolic fuel) and thus reduces sympathoadrenal (and other) responses to subsequent hypoglycemia.[3] Early findings were seemingly consistent with the idea of increased blood-to-brain transport of glucose, the primary brain metabolic fuel,[110] in the pathogenesis of HAAF. Hypoglycemia results in increased cerebral vascular expression of GLUT-1 and brain glucose uptake in rodents; however, that requires 3 days[111] or longer[112] of hypoglycemia, much longer than the <2 h of antecedent hypoglycemia known to reduce the sympathoadrenal response to subsequent hypoglycemia in humans.[30] Furthermore, brain glucose uptake, determined with the Kety-Schmidt technique, was reported to be maintained during hypoglycemia with prior hypoglycemia in individuals without diabetes and in patients with T1D with low A1C levels and, thus, likely recent antecedent hypoglycemia; however, in both instances,[113,114] the difference was greater estimated cerebral blood flows rather than increased glucose arteriovenous differences across the brain. Conversely, global blood-to-brain glucose transport, measured with [1-^{11}C]glucose PET, is not reduced in people with poorly controlled T1D,[59] and nearly 24 h of interprandial hypoglycemia (~55 mg/dL), which reduces the sympathoadrenal and symptomatic responses to subsequent hypoglycemia, does not increase global blood-to-brain glucose transport (or brain glucose metabolism) at the subphysiological plasma glucose concentration of 65 mg/dL (3.6 mmol/L) in healthy individuals.[115] Furthermore, global blood-to-brain [^{11}C]3-O-methylglucose[116] and [^{18}F]deoxyglucose[117,118] transport, both measured with PET, are not increased in patients with T1D with hypoglycemia unawareness. In addition, the rate of blood-to-brain glucose transport does not normally determine that of brain glucose metabolism; the former exceeds the latter even at slightly subphysiological plasma glucose concentrations.[59,115] As discussed in Chapter 2, the plasma glucose concentration at which glucose transport into the brain becomes limiting to brain glucose metabolism is <54 mg/dL (3.0 mmol/L).[119,120] An increase in blood-to-brain glucose transport during hypoglycemia would not be expected to increase brain glucose metabolism, and reduce the glucose counterregulatory response, unless transport were shifted from below to above that glycemic threshold. Furthermore, there was no difference in brain glucose concentrations in the individuals without diabetes and with T1D who were studied during euglycemia and hypoglycemia by van de Ven et al,[121] implying no difference in blood-to-brain glucose transport. These findings do not support the notion that increased blood-to-brain glucose transport is the mechanism of HAAF. If it is, the increase would need to be regional. The hypothesis, however, was based on global blood-to-brain glucose transport.[111–114] A variation on this theme would be increased glucose metabolism in the ventromedial hypothalamus in the absence of an increase in blood-to-brain glucose transport.[100,122–124] Given the finding that prior hypoglycemia did not increase global brain glucose metabolism in humans,[115] that mechanism also would need to be regional.

The brain, of course, can oxidize alternative fuels. Indeed, neurons normally oxidize lactate as well as glucose but that is largely lactate derived from glucose within the brain—mostly glucose transported from the circulation into the brain but partly that derived from glycogen in astrocytes.[125,126] A report of increased blood-to-brain acetate transport in patients with diabetes[127]—albeit not in patients with HAAF compared with those without HAAF—raised the possibility that increased transport of a monocarboxylate alternative fuel such as lactate might be involved in the pathogenesis of HAAF. Lactate infusions reduce epinephrine responses to, and symptoms of, hypoglycemia.[129,130] Plasma lactate concentrations roughly double during hyperinsulinemia.[20,24] Arteriovenous measurements have disclosed either no brain lactate uptake[131] or only a small brain lactate uptake[132] during hypoglycemia in humans, but lactate infusions have been shown to increase brain lactate uptake in individuals without diabetes[133,134] and to increase brain lactate concentrations in patients with T1D.[135] Indeed, it has been reported that antecedent hypoglycemia in nondiabetic rats results in an increase in lactate transport into the brain that provides only a modest increase in its contribution to total brain oxidative capacity but maintains brain glucose metabolism during subsequent hypoglycemia[136] and that lactate applied directly to the ventromedial hypothalamus increased hypothalamic γ-aminobutyrate (GABA), which inhibits the sympathoadrenal response to hypoglycemia.[137] Nonetheless, a simple lactate mechanism of HAAF has not evolved.[138]

Proton magnetic resonance spectroscopy disclosed less of a decrease in brain occipital lobe glutamate in patients with T1D with HAAF compared with patients without HAAF and individuals without diabetes.[139] The mechanism of that observation is not known, and any relevance to the pathogenesis of HAAF remains speculative.

The *brain metabolism hypothesis* posits that recent antecedent hypoglycemia (or sleep or prior exercise) alters the hypothalamic (and hind brain) regulation of the sympathoadrenal response to falling plasma glucose concentrations, resulting in HAAF.[3,100–102,140] Interestingly, this basically clinical issue—the mechanism of HAAF—has become a focus of fundamental neuroscience research probing the cellular and molecular mechanisms of the normal brain responses to hypoglycemia and the alterations that might lead to an attenuated sympathoadrenal response following episodes of hypoglycemia. Much of that focus has been on the ventromedial hypothalamus, a key site of the regulation of the sympathoadrenal response to falling glucose levels, and its glucose-excited and glucose-inhibited neurons. Potential mechanisms of the attenuated sympathoadrenal response to hypoglycemia include the following: *1*) decreased glucose sensing by glucose-excited or glucose-inhibited neurons in the hypothalamus, elsewhere in the brain and in the periphery; *2*) decreased activation of AMP kinase; *3*) increase glucokinase activity; *4*) loss of a decrease in the inhibitor GABA; *5*) loss of an increase in the stimulator glutamine; *6*) increased urocortin release; and *7*) reduced insulin action on the brain.

A variant of the brain metabolism hypothesis is the notion of brain glycogen supercompensation.[141] If the normally small astrocytic glycogen pool (see Chapter 2) increases substantially after hypoglycemia,[142] that expanded source of glucose (and lactate) within the brain could result in a reduced sympathoadrenal response during subsequent hypoglycemia. The evidence in rats that brain glycogen contents increase substantially above baseline after hypoglycemia[142] has not been confirmed[143,144] and the brain glycogen supercompensation hypothesis has not been supported in humans.[145] Brain glycogen contents were not increased in patients with T1D selected for hypoglycemia unawareness; if anything, they were lower than in controls. Parenthetically, that finding is also inconsistent with the thesis that an increase in blood-to-brain glucose transport causes HAAF. Because brain glycogen synthesis is a direct function of the plasma glucose concentration and blood-to-brain glucose transport, increased blood-to-brain glucose transport should result in increased brain glycogen; that was not the case in patients selected for HAAF.

Five potential pharmacological approaches to reversing HAAF—a selective serotonin reuptake inhibitor,[146–148] adrenergic antagonists,[98] an opioid receptor antagonist,[149,150] fructose[151] and a selective K_{ATP} channel agonist[152]—are of particular interest because they enhance glucose counterregulatory responses to falling plasma glucose concentrations—that is, the glucose counterregulatory responses become plasma glucose regulated, and they prevent the key feature of HAAF, the attenuated sympathoadrenal response to falling glucose levels.[3,153] Administration of a maximal dose of diazoxide has been reported to increase plasma catecholamine levels during hypoglycemia in patients with T1D.[154] A selective K_{ATP}, however, receptor agonist was found to further reduce, not increase, glucose counterregulatory responses to hypoglycemia in a model of HAAF in rats.[155]

Obviously, the brain metabolism and cerebral network hypotheses are not mutually exclusive because alterations in the former may well be components of the latter.

The emerging *cerebral network hypothesis* posits that recent antecedent hypoglycemia acts through a network of interconnected brain sites to inhibit hypothalamic activation and thus attenuate the sympathoadrenal response to subsequent hypoglycemia.[3,156,157] The concept is largely based on findings from neuroimaging of humans during hypoglycemia, particularly that with [^{15}O]water positron emission tomography ([^{15}O]water PET), which measures regional cerebral blood flow as an index of regional brain synaptic activity,[156–159] and the psychophysiological concept of habituation of the response to a given recurrent stress and its proposed mechanism. Hypothalamic-pituitary-adrenocortical (HPA) responses to a given stress, such as restraint stress, decrease after repeated exposures to that stress, a phenomenon termed habituation, in rats. The posterior paraventricular nucleus of the thalamus (PVNTh) is a brain site at which previous stress acts to modify responses to subsequent stress in rats.[160–163] Lesions of the PVNTh block habituation of the HPA response to repeated restraint.[161] Expression of the immediate early gene FosB has been reported to increase in the PVNTh, as well as in hypothalamic sites, during recurrent hypoglycemia in rats.[164] On the basis of measurements of plasma epinephrine and norepinephrine concentrations, habituation of the sympathoadrenal system response to repeated restraint stress also has been demonstrated in rats.[165,166]

Recent antecedent hypoglycemia has been shown to attenuate the sympathoadrenal response to subsequent hypoglycemia in humans without diabetes[30] and with diabetes.[17] That seems to be an example of habituation of the sympathoadrenal response in humans. Hypoglycemia has been found to increase synaptic activity in the thalamus, among other brain sites, by three investigative groups,[156,158,159,167] and to increase synaptic activity to a greater extent during hypoglycemia following recent antecedent hypoglycemia only in the dorsal midline thalamus, the site of the PVNTh (Figure 3.7).[156] Indeed, slightly subphysiological plasma glucose concentrations (e.g., 65 mg/dL, 3.5 mmol/L) increase dorsal midline thalamic synaptic activity selectively, or at least predominantly, in humans.[157] Thus, thalamic activation may be involved in the pathogenesis of the attenuated sympathoadrenal response to hypoglycemia that is the key feature of HAAF in diabetes.[3,156,157]

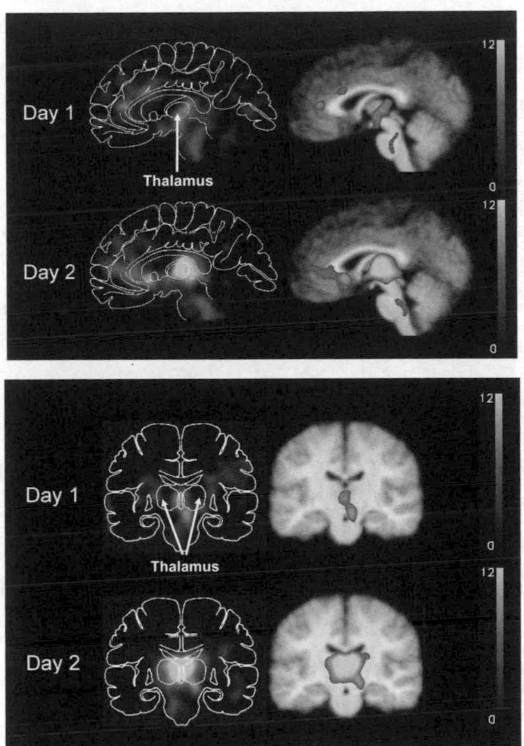

Figure 3.7—Increased dorsal midline thalamus synaptic activation, measured with ^{15}O water and positron emission tomography, in a model of HAAF in humans without diabetes.

Source: Reproduced from Arbeláez et al.[156] with permission from the American Diabetes Association.

Inactivation of the medial prefrontal cortex—by microinjection of the GABA-A receptor agonist muscimol—during recurrent restraint has been reported to prevent habituation of the HPA response to that stress in rats.[168] Increased synaptic activity in the medial prefrontal cortex (anterior cingulate) during hypoglycemia has been documented in humans.[156,158,159] Thus, the medial prefrontal cortex also may be involved in the cerebral network that results in the attenuated sympathoadrenal response to hypoglycemia that characterizes HAAF in diabetes. Brain sites in addition to the dorsal midline thalamus and the medial prefrontal cortex are undoubtedly involved.[156,158,159]

Cranston et al.[117] found a greater decrease in [^{18}F]deoxyglucose uptake in the subthalamic region of the brain, centered in the hypothalamus, during hypoglycemia in patients with T1D and hypoglycemia unawareness. That finding is consistent with the suggestion of increased thalamic inhibition of hypothalamic activity in HAAF.[156] The description of an array of differences in the patterns of [^{18}F]deoxyglucose uptake during hypoglycemia in patients with T1D with and without unawareness[117,118] is consistent with the participation of such a cerebral network in the pathogenesis of HAAF in diabetes.

Mechanisms of Hypoglycemic Death: Cardiovascular HAAF

Although we do not know precisely how often it kills people with diabetes, it is clear that hypoglycemia can kill[4,169] as discussed in detail in Chapter 1 (also see Figure 1.1). Estimates are that 2–10% of patients with T1D die from hypoglycemia.[170–177] Hypoglycemic deaths have been reported in many patients with T2D.[178–180]

Prolonged, profound hypoglycemia can cause brain death.[181–185] Neurons in the cerebral cortex and hippocampus are affected preferentially, followed by those in the basal ganglia and the thalamus in humans. The mechanism of brain death in experimental animals is thought to stem from increased glutamate release and sustained glutamate receptor activation when plasma glucose concentrations are <18 mg/dL (1.0 mmol/L), the EEG is isoelectric, and brain glucose and glycogen levels are unmeasurable. Steps in the pathway from glutamate receptor activation to neuron cell death include Ca^{2+} influx, mitochondrial calcium deregulation, production of reactive oxygen species, DNA damage, activation of poly(ADP-ribose polymerase-1 (PARP-1), mitochondrial permeability transition, and mitochondria-to-nucleus translocation of apoptosis-inducing factor.[182] PARP-1 inhibitors have been shown to reduce neuronal death.[186] It also has been reported that high blood glucose concentrations following experimental hypoglycemia can initiate neuronal death by a mechanism involving extracellular zinc release and activation of neuronal NADPH oxidase.[187] Such prolonged, profound hypoglycemia—with plasma glucose concentrations <18 mg/dL (1.0 mmol/L) and an isoelectric EEG—occurs rarely in patients with diabetes. Most fatal hypoglycemic episodes involve other mechanisms, presumably cardiac arrhythmias. Indeed, continuous interstitial glucose monitoring of patients with T2D disclosed higher rate of bradycardia (8.4-fold), atrial premature contractions (4.0-fold), and ventricular premature contractions (3.0-fold) during nocturnal hypoglycemia compared with euglycemia and have documented an association between hypoglycemia and ventricular arrhythmias in T2D.[188,189]

The mechanisms of such fatal hypoglycemic episodes have been reviewed.[3,169,190–196] These could include increased myocardial electrical vulnerability or vascular thrombosis. One cardiac mechanism is impaired ventricular repolarization, reflected in a prolonged corrected QT (QTc) interval in the electrocardiogram, which is known to be associated with lethal ventricular arrhythmias.[197] An association between the baseline QTc and cardiovascular mortality has been reported in T2D.[198] Epinephrine infusion increases the QTc interval.[199] Insulin-induced hypoglycemia, which causes catecholamine including epinephrine release, increases the QTc interval.[200] That effect is blunted by β-adrenergic antagonism with atenolol in people without diabetes[200] and in patients with T2D.[201] QTc interval prolongation occurs during spontaneous iatrogenic hypoglycemia in people with T1D[202–205] and those with T2D.[205–207] As mentioned, continuous electrocardiographic and subcutaneous glucose monitoring has disclosed atrial and ventricular contractions and periods of bradycardia during hypoglycemia in insulin-treated patients with T2D.[189,208] In addition, as a result of the cellular actions of insulin, and of released epinephrine, plasma potassium concentrations decline during insulin-induced hypoglycemia.[209] Such QTc interval prolongation and hypokalemia might occur in patients without or with ischemic heart disease or classical diabetic autonomic neuropathy (structural autonomic failure) or in those patients with cardiovascular HAAF (functional autonomic failure). With respect to the latter, compared with hyperinsulinemic euglycemia, hyperinsulinemic hypoglycemia was found to reduce baroreceptor sensitivity the following day in humans without diabetes[54,55] and with T1D.[55] That cardiovascular HAAF is entirely analogous to the metabolic HAAF discussed earlier in this chapter.

Given this background, the following concept of the pathogenesis of hypoglycemic mortality (see Figure 3.8) is plausible.[4,169] Recent antecedent hypoglycemia causes cardiovascular HAAF, including reduced baroreflex sensitivity and the resulting increased vulnerability to a ventricular arrhythmia. Recent antecedent hypoglycemia also causes metabolic HAAF with an increased risk for an episode of iatrogenic hypoglycemia with sympathoadrenal activation

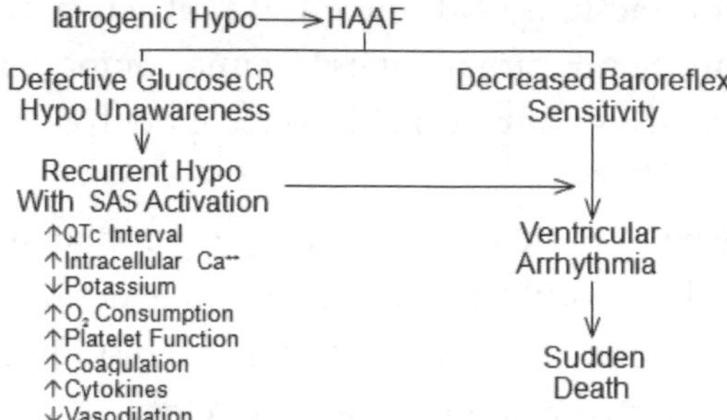

Figure 3.8—Potential mechanism of iatrogenic hypoglycemia–induced hypoglycemia-associated autonomic failure (HAAF)–mediated sudden death in diabetes: cardiovascular HAAF causing reduced baroreceptor sensitivity and metabolic HAAF causing defective glucose counterregulation (CR) and hypoglycemia (Hypo) unawareness and leading to an episode of hypoglycemia that increases sympathoadrenal system (SAS) activity, which triggers a fatal ventricular arrhythmia in the setting of reduced baroreflex sensitivity.

Source: From Cryer[169] with permission from the American Journal of Medicine.

that could, in the setting of decreased baroreflex sensitivity and through an array of mechanisms including abnormal cardiac repolarization, trigger a ventricular arrhythmia and sudden death. Experimental data support the role of a sympathoadrenal discharge in that both CNS glucose infusion and β-adrenergic blockade reduced deaths of rats during marked hypoglycemia.[210]

Is HAAF Adaptive or Maladaptive?

As discussed in this chapter, recent antecedent iatrogenic hypoglycemia shifts glycemic thresholds to lower levels and attenuates sympathoadrenal and symptomatic responses at a given level of subsequent hypoglycemia[17,30] and thus causes HAAF in diabetes.[3] HAAF increases the risk of severe iatrogenic hypoglycemia during intensive therapy of diabetes.[37,38] Severe hypoglycemia is associated with arrhythmic death in patients with diabetes,[189,211] and during marked hypoglycemia in rodents, mortality is mediated by sympathoadrenal activation. This activation commonly results in progressive atrioventricular block and terminal bradycardia, which are prevented by β-adrenergic antagonism and reduced by recent antecedent hypoglycemia in nondiabetic and diabetic rats.[210,212] Furthermore, mortality in patients with diabetes appears to some extent to be conversely related to the frequency of hypoglycemia.[213,214] These findings suggest that HAAF in diabetes is both maladaptive—in that it increases the risk of iatrogenic hypoglycemia, may increase the risk of hypoglycemic death, and might contribute to the pathogenesis of arteriosclerotic disease—and adaptive—in that it decreases the frequency of hypoglycemia death.[215] Both of these phenomena are plausibly attributable to a decreased sympathoadrenal response to a given level of hypoglycemia, largely the result of recent antecedent iatrogenic hypoglycemia. That does not, of course, exclude a vigorous and potentially lethal sympathoadrenal response to more marked hypoglycemia.

Summary

Insulin excess of sufficient magnitude can cause iatrogenic hypoglycemia. In the vast majority of instances, however, it is the integrity of physiological and behavioral defenses against falling plasma glucose concentrations that determines whether an episode of relative, or even absolute, therapeutic hyperinsulinemia results in an episode of hypoglycemia. Thus, hypoglycemia is typically the result of the interplay of therapeutic insulin excess and compromised glycemic defenses (i.e., HAAF) in T1D and advanced T2D. The common denominator of the two components of HAAF—defective glucose counterregulation and hypoglycemia unawareness—is an attenuated sympathoadrenal response to a given level of hypoglycemia. In addition to therapeutic hyperinsulinemia, absent decrements in insulin and absent increments in glucagon, both the result of β-cell failure in T1D and advanced T2D, are prerequisites for defective glucose counterregulation. In that setting, attenuated epinephrine responses cause that clinical syndrome. Attenuated sympathoadrenal responses, largely reduced sympathetic neural responses, also cause the clinical syndrome of hypoglycemia unawareness. The attenuated sympathoadrenal responses, the key feature of HAAF, can be caused by recent antecedent hypoglycemia, prior exercise, or sleep, among other causes. The fact that loss of the insulin and glucagon responses stems from β-cell failure explains why HAAF develops early in the course of T1D but only later in the course of T2D. That development, in turn, explains why iatrogenic hypoglycemia becomes limiting to glycemic control early in T1D but later in T2D. Decreased baroreflex sensitivity, a feature of cardiovascular HAAF, may set the stage for a fatal ventricular arrhythmia triggered by the sympathoadrenal response to a subsequent episode of hypoglycemia, the result of metabolic HAAF. Finally, it is conceivable that HAAF both makes patients with diabetes more prone to recurrent hypoglycemia and less vulnerable to the devastating effects of hypoglycemia.

Understanding this pathophysiology of glucose counterregulation in diabetes leads directly to insight into the risk factors for (see Chapter 4), the definition and classification of (see Chapter 5), and the prevention or treatment of (see Chapter 6) clinical iatrogenic hypoglycemia in diabetes.

References

1. Cryer PE. Diverse causes of hypoglycemia-associated autonomic failure in diabetes. *N Engl J Med* 2004;350:2272–2279
2. Cryer PE. The barrier of hypoglycemia in diabetes. *Diabetes* 2008;57:3169–3176
3. Cryer PE. Mechanisms of hypoglycemia-associated autonomic failure in diabetes. *N Engl J Med* 2013;369:362–372
4. Cryer PE. Glycemic goals in diabetes: trade-off between glycemic control and iatrogenic hypoglycemia. *Diabetes* 2014;63:2188–2195
5. Cryer PE. Hypoglycemia in diabetes. In *Textbook of Diabetes,* 4th ed. Holt RIG, Cockram C, Flyvbjerg A, Goldstein BJ, Eds. Oxford, U.K., Wiley-Blackwell, 2010, p. 528–545
6. Cryer PE. Hypoglycemia. In *Williams Textbook of Endocrinology*. 13th ed. Melmed S, Polonsky KS, Larsen PR, Kronenberg HM, Eds. Philadelphia, Elsevier, 2016, p. 1582–1607.
7. Turner RC, Cull CA, Frighi V, Holman RR, U.K. Prospective Diabetes Study (UKPDS) Group. Glycemic control with diet, sulfonylurea, metformin, or insulin in patients with type 2 diabetes mellitus: progressive requirement for multiple therapies (UKPDS 49). *JAMA* 1999;281:2005–2012
8. Bolen S, Feldman L, Vassy J, Wilson L, Yeh HC, Marinopoulos S, Wiley C, Selvin E, Wilson R, Bass E, Brancati FL. Systemic review: comparative effective-

ness and safety of oral medications for type 2 diabetes mellitus. *Ann Intern Med* 2007;147:386–399

9. Phung OJ, Scholle JM, Talwar M, Coleman CL. Effect of noninsulin antidiabetic drugs added to metformin therapy on glycemic control, weight gain, and hypoglycemia in type 2 diabetes. *JAMA* 2010;303:1410–1418

10. Tschope D, Bramlage P, Binz C, Krekler M, Plate T, Deeg E, Gitt AK. Antidiabetic pharmacotherapy and anamnestic hypoglycemia in a large cohort of type 2 diabetic patients an analysis of the DiaRegis registry. *Cardiovasc Diabetol* 2011;10:66

11. Ferrannini E, Ramos SJ, Salsali A, Tang W, List JF. Dapagliflozin monotherapy in type 2 diabetic patients with inadequate glycemic control by diet and exercise. A randomized, double-blind, placebo-controlled, phase 3 trial. *Diabetes Care* 2010;33:2217–2224

12. U.K. Prospective Diabetes Study Group (UKPDS). Overview of 6 years of therapy of type II diabetes: a progressive disease. *Diabetes* 1995;44:1249–1258

13. Wright AD, Cull CA, MacLeod KM, Holman RR, for the UKPDS Group. Hypoglycemia in type 2 diabetic patients randomized to and maintained on monotherapy with diet, sulfonylurea, metformin, or insulin for 6 years from diagnosis: UKPDS 73. *J Diabetes Complications* 2006;20:395–401

14. U.K. Hypoglycaemia Study Group (UK Hypo Group). Risk of hypoglycaemia in types 1 and 2 diabetes: effects of treatment modalities and their duration. *Diabetologia* 2007;50:1140–1147

15. Cryer PE. The prevention and correction of hypoglycemia. In *Handbook of Physiology.* Section 7, The Endocrine System. Vol. II, The Endocrine Pancreas and Regulation of Metabolism. Jefferson LS, Cherrington AD, Eds. New York, Oxford University Press, 2001, p. 1057–1092

16. DeRosa MA, Cryer PE. Hypoglycemia and the sympathoadrenal system: neurogenic symptoms are largely the result of sympathetic neural, rather than adrenomedullary, activation. *Am J Physiol Endocrinol Metab* 2004;287:E32–E41

17. Dagogo-Jack SE, Craft S, Cryer PE. Hypoglycemia-associated autonomic failure in insulin-dependent diabetes mellitus. *J Clin Invest* 1993;91:819–828

18. Segel SA, Paramore DS, Cryer PE. Hypoglycemia-associated autonomic failure in advanced type 2 diabetes. *Diabetes* 2002;51:724–733

19. Banarer S, McGregor VP, Cryer PE. Intraislet hyperinsulinemia prevents the glucagon response to hypoglycemia despite an intact autonomic response. *Diabetes* 2002;51:958–965

20. Raju B, Cryer PE. Loss of the decrement in intraislet insulin plausibly explains loss of the glucagon response to hypoglycemia in insulin-deficient diabetes. *Diabetes* 2005;54:757–764

21. Gosmanov NR, Szoke E, Israelian Z, Smith T, Cryer PE, Gerich JE, Meyer C. Role of the decrement in intraislet insulin for the glucagon response to hypoglycemia in humans. *Diabetes Care* 2005;28:1124–1131

22. Israelian Z, Gosmanov NR, Szoke E, Schorr M, Bokhari S, Cryer PE, Gerich JE, Meyer C. Increasing the decrement in intraislet insulin improves glucagon responses to hypoglycemia in advanced type 2 diabetes. *Diabetes Care* 2005;28: 2691–2696

23. Cooperberg BA, Cryer PE. β-cell-mediated signaling predominates over direct α-cell signaling in the regulation of glucagon secretion in humans. *Diabetes Care* 2009;32:2275–2280

24. Cooperberg BA, Cryer PE. Insulin reciprocally regulates glucagon secretion in humans. *Diabetes* 2010;59:2936–2940

25. Cryer PE. Glucagon in the pathogenesis of hypoglycemia and hyperglycemia in diabetes. *Endocrinology* 2012;153:1039–1048

26. Gerich JE, Langlois M, Noacco C, Karam J, Forsham P. Lack of glucagon response to hypoglycemia in diabetes: evidence for an intrinsic pancreatic alpha-cell defect. *Science* 1973;182:171–173

27. Bolli G, De Feo P, Compagnucci P, Cartechini MG, Angeletti F, Santeusanio F, Brunetti P, Gerich JE. Abnormal glucose counterregulation in insulin dependent diabetes: interaction of anti-insulin antibodies and impaired glucagon and epinephrine secretion. *Diabetes* 1983;32:134–141

28. Cryer PE. Mechanisms of hypoglycemia-associated autonomic failure and its component syndromes in diabetes. *Diabetes* 2005;54:3592–3601

29. Cryer PE. Hypoglycaemia: the limiting factor in the glycaemic management of the critically ill? *Diabetologia* 2006;49:1722–1725

30. Heller SR, Cryer PE. Reduced neuroendocrine and symptomatic responses to subsequent hypoglycemia after one episode of hypoglycemia in nondiabetic humans. *Diabetes* 1991;40:223–226

31. Galassetti P, Mann S, Tate D, Neill RA, Costa F, Wasserman DH, Davis SN. Effects of antecedent prolonged exercise on subsequent counterregulatory responses to hypoglycemia. *Am J Physiol Endocrinol Metab* 2001;280:E908–E917

32. Sandoval DA, Aftab Guy DL, Richardson MA, Ertl AC, Davis SN. Effects of low and moderate antecedent exercise on counterregulatory responses to subsequent hypoglycemia in type 1 diabetes. *Diabetes* 2004;53:1798–1806

33. Ertl AC, Davis SN. Evidence for a vicious cycle of exercise and hypoglycemia in type 1 diabetes mellitus. *Diabetes Metab Res Rev* 2004;20:124–130

34. Jones TW, Porter P, Sherwin RS, Davis EA, O'Leary P, Frazer F, Byrne G, Stick S, Tamborlane WV. Decreased epinephrine responses to hypoglycemia during sleep. *N Engl J Med* 1998;338:1657–1662

35. Banarer S, Cryer PE. Sleep-related hypoglycemia-associated autonomic failure in type 1 diabetes. Reduced awakening from sleep during hypoglycemia. *Diabetes* 2003;52:1195–1203

36. Schultes B, Jauch-Chara K, Gais S, Hallschmid M, Reiprich E, Kern W, Oltmanns KM, Peters A, Fehm HL, Born J. Defective awakening response to nocturnal hypoglycemia in patients with type 1 diabetes mellitus. *PLoS Medicine* 2007;4:e69

37. White NH, Skor DA, Cryer PE, Levandoski LA, Bier DM, Santiago JV. Identification of type 1 diabetic patients at increased risk for hypoglycemia during intensive therapy. *N Engl J Med* 1983;308:485–491

38. Bolli GB, De Feo P, De Cosmo S, Perriello G, Ventura MM, Massi-Benedetti M, Santeusanio F, Gerich JE, Brunetti P. A reliable and reproducible test for adequate glucose counter-regulation in type 1 diabetes mellitus. *Diabetes* 1984;33:732–737

39. Ly TT, Gallego PH, Davis EA, Jones TW. Impaired awareness of hypoglycemia in a population-based sample of children and adolescents with type 1 diabetes. *Diabetes Care* 2009;32:1802–1806

40. Giménez M, Lara M, Jiménez A, Conget I. Glycemic profile characteristics and frequency of impaired awareness of hypoglycaemia in subjects with T1D and repeated hypoglycaemic events. *Acta Diabetol* 2009;46:291–293

41. Geddes J, Schopman JE, Zammitt NN, Frier BM. Prevalence of impaired awareness of hypoglycaemia in adults with type 1 diabetes. *Diabet Med* 2008;25:501–504

42. Schopman JE, Geddes J, Frier BM. Prevalence of impaired awareness of hypoglycaemia and frequency of hypoglycaemia in insulin-treated type 2 diabetes. *Diabetes Res Clin Pract* 2010;87:64–68

43. Schopman JE, Geddes J, Frier BM. Frequency of symptomatic and asymptomatic hypoglycaemia in type 1 diabetes: effect of impaired awareness of hypoglycaemia. *Diabet Med* 2011;28:352–355

44. Sejling AS, Kjaer TW, Pedersen-Bjergaard U, Diemar SS, Frandsen CS, Hilsted L, Faber J, Holst JJ, Tarnow L, Nielsen MN, Remvig LS, Thorsteinsson B, Juhl CB. Hypoglycemia-associated changes in the electroencephalogram in patients with type 1 diabetes and normal hypoglycemia awareness or unawareness. *Diabetes* 2015;64:1760–1769

45. Berlin I, Grimaldi A, Payan C, Sachon C, Bosquet F, Thervet F, Puech AJ. Hypoglycemic symptoms and decreased β-adrenergic sensitivity in insulin dependent diabetic patients. *Diabetes Care* 1987;10:742–747

46. Fritsche A, Stefan N, Häring H, Gerich J, Stumvoll M. Avoidance of hypoglycemia restores hypoglycemia awareness by increasing β-adrenergic sensitivity in type 1 diabetes. *Ann Intern Med* 2001;134:729–736

47. de Galan BE, De Mol P, Wennekes L, Schouwenberg BJJ, Smits P. Preserved sensitivity to β2-adrenergic receptor agonists in patients with type 1 diabetes mellitus and hypoglycemia unawareness. *J Clin Endocrinol Metab* 2006;91:2878–2881

48. Schouwenberg BJJ, Smits P, Tack CJ, de Galan BE. The effect of antecedent hypoglycaemia on β_2-adrenergic sensitivity in healthy participants with the Arg16Gly polymorphism of the β_2-adrenergic receptor. *Diabetologia* 2011;54:1212–1218

49. Cryer PE. Iatrogenic hypoglycemia as a cause of hypoglycemia-associated autonomic failure in IDDM: a vicious cycle. *Diabetes* 1992;41:255–260

50. Cryer PE. Mechanisms of sympathoadrenal failure and hypoglycemia in diabetes. *J Clin Invest* 2006;116:1470–1473

51. Ryder REJ, Owens DR, Hayes TM, Ghatei MA, Bloom SR. Unawareness of hypoglycaemia and inadequate hypoglycaemic counterregulation: no causal relation with diabetic autonomic neuropathy. *BMJ* 1990;301:783–787

52. Bottini P, Boschetti E, Pampanelli S, Ciofetta M, Del Sindaco P, Scionti L, Brunetti P, Bolli GB. Contribution of autonomic neuropathy to reduced plasma adrenaline responses to hypoglycemia in IDDM. Evidence for a nonselective defect. *Diabetes* 1997;46:814–823

53. Meyer C, Grossman R, Mitrakou A, Mahler R, Veneman T, Gerich J, Bretzel RG. Effects of autonomic neuropathy on counterregulation and awareness of hypoglycemia in type 1 diabetic patients. *Diabetes Care* 1998;21:1960–1966

54. Adler GK, Bonyhay I, Failing H, Waring E, Dotson S, Freeman R. Antecedent hypoglycemia impairs cardiovascular function. Implications for rigorous glycemic control. *Diabetes* 2009;58:360–366

55. Limberg JK, Farni KE, Taylor JL, Dube S, Basu A, Basu R, Wehrwein EA, Joyner MJ. Autonomic control during acute hypoglycemia in type 1 diabetes mellitus. *Clin Auton Res* 2014;24:275–283

56. Dagogo-Jack S, Rattarasarn C, Cryer PE. Reversal of hypoglycemia unawareness, but not defective glucose counterregulation, in IDDM. *Diabetes* 1994;43:1426–1434

57. Fanelli CG, Epifano L, Rambotti AM, Pampanelli S, Di Vincenzo A, Modarelli F, Lepore M, Annibale B, Ciofetta M, Bottini P, Porcellati F, Scionti L, Santeusanio F, Brunetti P, Bolli GB. Meticulous prevention of hypoglycemia normalizes the glycemic thresholds and magnitude of most of neuroendocrine responses to, symptoms of, and cognitive function during hypoglycemia in intensively treated patients with short-term IDDM. *Diabetes* 1993;42:1683–1689

58. Fanelli C, Pampanelli S, Epifano L, Rambotti AM, Di Vincenzo A, Modarelli F, Ciofetta M, Lepore M, Annibale B, Torlone E, Perriello G, De Feo P, Santeusanio F, Brunetti P, Bolli GB. Long-term recovery from unawareness, deficient counterregulation and lack of cognitive dysfunction during hypoglycemia, following institution of rational, intensive therapy in IDDM. *Diabetologia* 1994;37:1265–1276

59. Fanelli CG, Dence CS, Markham J, Videen TO, Paramore DS, Cryer PE, Powers WJ. Blood-to-brain glucose transport and cerebral glucose metabolism are not reduced in poorly controlled type 1 diabetes. *Diabetes* 1998;47:1444–1450

60. Ovalle F, Fanelli CG, Paramore DS, Hershey T, Craft S, Cryer PE. Brief twice-weekly episodes of hypoglycemia reduce detection of clinical hypoglycemia in type 1 diabetes mellitus. *Diabetes* 1998;47:1472–1479

61. Cranston I, Lomas J, Maran A, Macdonald I, Amiel SA. Restoration of hypoglycaemia awareness in patients with long-duration insulin-dependent diabetes. *Lancet* 1994;344:283–287

62. Ang M, Meyer C, Brendel MD, Bretzel RG, Linn T. Magnitude and mechanisms of glucose counterregulation following islet transplantation in patients with type 1 diabetes suffering from severe hypoglycaemic episodes. *Diabetologia* 2014;57:623–632

63. Rickels MR, Fuller C, Dalton-Bakes C, Markmann E, Palanjian M, Cullison K, Yiao J, Kapoor S, Liu C, Naji A, Teff KL. Restoration of glucose counterregulation by islet transplantation in long-standing type 1 diabetes. *Diabetes* 2015;64:1713–1718

64. Davis SN, Mann S, Briscoe VJ, Ertl AC, Tate DB. Effects of intensive therapy and antecedent hypoglycemia on counterregulatory responses to hypoglycemia in type 2 diabetes. *Diabetes* 2009;58:701–709

65. Spyer G, Hattersley AT, Macdonald IA, Amiel S, MacLeod KM. Hypoglycaemic counter-regulation at normal blood glucose concentrations in patients with well controlled type-2 diabetes. *Lancet* 2000;356:1970–1974

66. Levy CJ, Kinsley BT, Bajaj M, Simonson DC. Effect of glycemic control on glucose counterregulation during hypoglycemia in NIDDM. *Diabetes Care* 1998;21: 1330–1338

67. Choudhary P, Lonnen K, Emery CJ, MacDonald IA, MacLeod KM, Amiel SA, Heller SR. Comparing hormonal and symptomatic responses to experimental hypoglycaemia in insulin- and sulfonylurea-treated type 2 diabetes. *Diabet Med* 2009;26:665–672

68. Amiel SA, Sherwin RS, Simonson DC, Tamborlane WV. Effect of intensive insulin therapy on glycemic thresholds for counterregulatory hormone release. *Diabetes* 1988;37:901–907

69. Boyle PJ, Schwartz NS, Shah SD, Clutter WE, Cryer PE. Plasma glucose concentrations at the onset of hypoglycemic symptoms in patients with poorly controlled diabetes and in nondiabetics. *N Engl J Med* 1988;318:1487–1492

70. Tansey MJ, Tsalikian E, Beck RW, Mauras N, Buckingham BA, Weinzimer SA, Janz KF, Kollman C, Xing D, Ruedy KJ, Steffes MW, Borland TM, Singh RJ, Tamborlane WV, for the Diabetes Research in Children Network (DirecNet) Study Group. The effects of aerobic exercise on glucose and counterregulatory hormone concentrations in children with type 1 diabetes. *Diabetes Care* 2006;29:20–25

71. Ruegemer JJ, Squires RW, Marsh HM, Haymond MW, Cryer PE, Rizza RA, Miles JM. Differences between prebreakfast and late afternoon glycemic responses to exercise in IDDM patients. *Diabetes Care* 1990;13:104–110

72. MacDonald MJ. Post exercise late onset hypoglycemia in insulin-dependent diabetic patients. *Diabetes Care* 1987;10:584–588

73. Tsalikian E, Mauras N, Beck RW, Tamborlane WV, Janz KF, Chase HP, Wysocki T, Weinzimer SA, Buckingham BA, Kollman C, Xing D, Ruedy KJ, for the Diabetes Research in Network (DirecNet) Study Group. Impact of exercise on overnight glycemic control in children with type 1 diabetes. *J Pediatr* 2005;147: 528–534

74. Metcalf KM, Singhvi A, Tsalikian E, Tansey MJ, Zimmerman MB, Esliger DW, Janz KF. Effects of moderate-to-vigorous intensity physical activity on overnight and next-day hypoglycemia in active adolescents with type 1 diabetes. *Diabetes Care* 2014;37:1272–1278

75. Younk LM, Davis SN. Hypoglycemia and hypoglycemia unawareness during and following exercise in type 1 diabetes. *In Type 1 Diabetes:Clinical Management of the Athlete.* Gallen I, Ed. London, Springer-Verlag, 2012. p. 155–150

76. Raju B, Arbeláez AM, Breckenridge SM, Cryer PE. Nocturnal hypoglycemia in type 1 diabetes: an assessment of preventive bedtime treatments. *J Clin Endocrinol Metab* 2006;91:2087–2092

77. Jennum P, Stender-Petersen K, Rabøl R, Jørgensen NR, Chu PL, Madsbad S. The impact of nocturnal hypoglycemia on sleep in subjects with type 2 diabetes. *Diabetes Care* 201538:2151–2157

78. Yun J-S, Kim J-H, Song K-H, Ahn Y-B, Yoon K-H, Yoo K-D, Park Y-M, Ko S-H. Cardiovascular autonomic dysfunction predicts severe hypoglycemia in patients with type 2 diabetes: a 10-year follow-up study. *Diabetes Care* 2014; 37:235–241

79. de Galan BE, Tack CJ, Willemsen JJ, Sweep CGJ, Smits P, Lenders JWM. Plasma metanephrine levels are decreased in type 1 diabetic patients with a severely impaired epinephrine response to hypoglycemia, indicating reduced stores of epinephrine. *J Clin Endocrinol Metab* 2004;89:2057–2061

80. Arbeláez AM, Xing D, Cryer PE, Kollman C, Beck RW, Sherr J, Ruedy KJ, Tamborlane WV, Mauras N, Tsalikian E, Wilson DM, White NH, for the Diabetes Research in Children Network (DirecNet) Study Group. Blunted glucagon but not epinephrine responses to hypoglycemia occurs in youth with less than 1 yr duration of type 1 diabetes mellitus. *Pediatr Diabetes* 2014;15: 127–134

81. Wiethop BV, Cryer PE. Glycemic actions of alanine and terbutaline in IDDM. *Diabetes Care* 1993;16:1124–1130

82. Caprio S, Tamborlane WV, Zych K, Gerow K, Sherwin RS. Loss of potentiating effect of hypoglycemia on the glucagon response to hyperaminoacidemia in IDDM. *Diabetes* 1993;42:550–555

83. Hoffman RP, Singer-Granick C, Drash AL, Becker DJ. Abnormal alpha cell hypoglycemic recognition in children with insulin dependent diabetes mellitus (IDDM). *J Pediatr Endocrinol* 1994;7:225–234

84. Rossetti P, Porcellati F, Busciantella Ricci N, Candeloro P, Cioli P, Nair KS, Santeusanio F, Bolli GB, Fanelli CG. Effect of oral amino acids on counterregulatory responses and cognitive function during insulin-induced hypoglycemia in nondiabetic and type 1 diabetic people. *Diabetes* 2008;57:1905–1917

85. Fukuda M, Tanaka A, Tahara Y, Ikegami H, Yamamoto Y, Kumahara Y, Shima K. Correlation between minimal secretory capacity of pancreatic β-cells and stability of diabetic control. *Diabetes* 1988;37:81–88

86. Menge BA, Grüber L, Jørgensen SM, Deacon CF, Schmidt WE, Veldhuis JD, Holst JJ, Meier JJ. Loss of inverse relationship between pulsatile insulin and glucagon secretion in patients with type 2 diabetes. *Diabetes* 2011;60:2160–2168

87. Taborsky GJ Jr, Mei Q, Hackney DJ, Figlewicz DP, LeBoeuf R, Mundinger TO. Loss of islet sympathetic nerves and impairment of glucagon secretion in the NOD mouse: relationship to invasive insulitis. *Diabetologia* 2009;52:2602–2611

88. McCrimmon RY, Sherwin RS. Hypoglycemia in type 1 diabetes. *Diabetes* 2010;59:2333–2339

89. Diem P, Redmon JB, Abid M, Moran A, Sutherland DER, Halter JB, Robertson RP. Glucagon, catecholamine and pancreatic polypeptide secretion in type 1 diabetic recipients of pancreatic allografts. *J Clin Invest* 1990;86:2008–2013

90. Sherck SM, Shiota M, Saccomando J, Cardin S, Allen EJ, Hastings JR, Neal DW, Williams PE, Cherrington AD. Pancreatic response to mild non-insulin induced hypoglycemia does not involve extrinsic neural input. *Diabetes* 2001;50:2487–2496

91. Palmer JP, Henry DP, Benson JW, Johnson DG, Ensinck JW. Glucagon response to hypoglycemia in sympathectomized man. *J Clin Invest* 1976;57:522–525

92. Gerich JE, Charles MA, Grodsky GM. Characterization of the effects of arginine and glucose on glucagon and insulin release from the perfused rat pancreas. *J Clin Invest* 1974;54:833–841

93. Walker JN, Ramracheya R, Zhang Q, Johnson PRV, Braun M, Rorsman P. Regulation of glucagon secretion by glucose: paracrine, intrinsic or both? *Diabetes Obes Metab* 2011;13(Suppl. 1):95–105

94. Rizza RA, Cryer PE, Gerich JE. Role of glucagon, catecholamines, and growth hormone in human glucose counterregulation. *J Clin Invest* 1979;64:62–71

95. Yue JT, Burdett E, Coy DH, Giacca A, Efendic S, Vranic M. Somatostatin receptor type 2 antagonism improves glucagon and corticosterone counterregulatory responses to hypoglycemia in streptozotocin-induced diabetic rats. *Diabetes* 2012;61:197–207

96. Yue JT, Riddell MC, Burdett E, Coy DH, Efendic S, Vranic M. Amelioration of hypoglycemia via somatostatin receptor type 2 antagonism in recurrently hypoglycemic diabetic rats. *Diabetes* 2013;62:2215–2222

97. Karimian N, Qin T, Liang T, Osundiji M, Huang Y, Teich T, Riddell MC, Cattral MS, Coy DH, Vranic M, Gaisano HY. Somatostatin receptor type 2 antagonism improves glucagon counterregulation in biobreeding diabetic rats. *Diabetes* 2013;62:2968–2977

98. Ramanathan RP, Cryer PE. Adrenergic mediation of hypoglycemia-associated autonomic failure. *Diabetes* 2011;60:602–606

99. Szepietowska B, Zhu W, Chan O, Horblitt A, Dziura J, Sherwin RS. Modulation of β-adrenergic receptors in the ventromedial hypothalamus influences counterregulatory responses to hypoglycemia. *Diabetes* 2011;60:3154–3158

100. Levin BE, Becker TC, Eiki J, Zhang BB, Dunn-Meynell AA. Ventromedial hypothalamic glucokinase is an important mediator of the counterregulatory response to insulin-induced hypoglycemia. *Diabetes* 2008;57:1371–1379

101. Beall C, Ashford ML, McCrimmon RJ. The physiology and pathophysiology of the neural control of the counterregulatory response. *Am J Physiol Regul Integr Comp Physiol* 2012;302:R215–R223

102. Chan O, Sherwin R. Influence of VMH fuel sensing on hypoglycemic responses. *Trends Endocrinol Metab* 2013;24:616–624

103. Davis SN, Shavers C, Costa F, Mosqueda-Garcia R. Role of cortisol in the pathogenesis of deficient counterregulation after antecedent hypoglycemia in normal humans. *J Clin Invest* 1996;98:680–691

104. Davis SN, Shavers C, Davis B, Costa F. Prevention of an increase in plasma cortisol during hypoglycemia preserves subsequent counterregulatory responses. *J Clin Invest* 1997;100:429–438

105. McGregor VP, Banarer S, Cryer PE. Elevated endogenous cortisol reduces autonomic neuroendocrine and symptom responses to subsequent hypoglycemia. *Am J Physiol Endocrinol Metab* 2002;282:E770–E777

106. Raju B, McGregor VP, Cryer PE. Cortisol elevations comparable to those that occur during hypoglycemia do not cause hypoglycemia-associated autonomic failure. *Diabetes* 2003;52:2083–2089

107. Goldberg PA, Weiss R, McCrimmon RJ, Hintz EV, Dziura J, Sherwin RS. Antecedent hypercortisolemia is not primarily responsible for generating hypoglycemia-associated autonomic failure. *Diabetes* 2006;55:1121–1126

108. Bao S, Briscoe VJ, Tate DB, Davis SN. Effects of differing antecedent increases of plasma cortisol on counterregulatory responses during subsequent exercise in type 1 diabetes. *Diabetes* 2009;58:2100–2108

109. de Galan BE, Rietjens SJ, Tack CJ, Van der Werf SP, Sweep CGJ, Lenders JWM, Smits P. Antecedent adrenaline attenuates the responsiveness to, but not the release of, counterregulatory hormones during subsequent hypoglycemia. *J Clin Endocrinol Metab* 2003;88:5462–5467

110. Clarke DD, Sokoloff L. Circulation and energy metabolism of the brain. In *Basic Neurochemistry: Molecular, Cellular and Medical Aspects.* 5th ed. Siegel G, Agranoff B, Albers RW, Molinoff P, Eds. New York, Raven Press, 1994, p. 645–680

111. McCall AL, Fixman LB, Fleming N, Tornheim K, Chick W, Ruderman NB. Chronic hypoglycemia increases brain glucose transport. *Am J Physiol* 1986;251: E442–E447

112. Simpson IA, Appel NM, Hokari M, Oki J, Holman GD, Maher F, Koehler-Stec EM, Vannucci SJ, Smith QR. Blood-brain barrier glucose transporter: effects of hypo- and hyperglycemia revisited. *J Neurochem* 1999;72:238–247

113. Boyle PJ, Nagy RJ, O'Connor AM, Kempers SF, Yeo RA, Qualls C. Adaptation in brain glucose uptake following recurrent hypoglycemia. *Proc Natl Acad Sci USA* 1994;91:9352–9356

114. Boyle PJ, Kempers SF, O'Connor AM, Nagy RJ. Brain glucose uptake and unawareness of hypoglycemia in patients with insulin dependent diabetes mellitus. *N Engl J Med* 1995;333:1726–1731

115. Segel SA, Fanelli CG, Dence CS, Markham J, Videen TO, Paramore DS, Powers WJ, Cryer PE. Blood-to-brain glucose transport, cerebral glucose metabolism and cerebral blood flow are not increased following hypoglycemia. *Diabetes* 2001;50:1911–1917

116. Bingham EM, Dunn JT, Smith D, Sutcliffe-Goulden J, Reed LJ, Marsden PK, Amiel SA. Differential changes in brain glucose metabolism during hypoglycaemia accompany loss of hypoglycaemia awareness in men with type 1 diabetes mellitus. An [^{11}C]-3-O-methyl-D-glucose PET study. *Diabetologia* 2005;48: 2080–2089

117. Cranston I, Reed LJ, Marsden PK, Amiel SA. Changes in regional brain ^{18}F-fluorodeoxyglucose uptake at hypoglycemia in type 1 diabetic men associated with hypoglycemia unawareness and counter-regulatory failure. *Diabetes* 2001; 50:2329–2336

118. Dunn JT, Cranston I, Marsden PK, Amiel SA, Reed LJ. Attenuation of amygdala and frontal cortical responses to low blood glucose concentration in asymptomatic hypoglycemia in type 1 diabetes. *Diabetes* 2007;56:2766–2773

119. van de Ven KCC, de Galan BE, van der Graaf M, Shestov AA, Henry P-G, Tack CJJ, Heerschap A. Effect of acute hypoglycemia on human cerebral glucose metabolism measured by ^{13}C magnetic resonance spectroscopy. *Diabetes* 2011;60:1467–1473

120. Antenor-Dorsey JAV, Khoury N, Su Y, Shackleford AM, Jethi KG, Powers WJ, Cryer PE, Arbeláez AM. The adrenomedullary epinephrine response to declining plasma glucose concentrations is a signaling event that is not caused by a decrease in the cerebral metabolic rate of glucose (abstract). *Diabetes* 2013; 62:A100

121. van de Ven KC, van der Graaf M, Tack CJ, Heerschap A, de Galan BE. Steady-state brain glucose concentrations during hypoglycemia in healthy humans and patients with type 1 diabetes. *Diabetes* 2012;61:1974–1977

122. Kang L, Sanders NM, Dunn-Meynell AA, Gaspers LD, Routh VH, Thomas AP, Levin BE. Prior hypoglycemia enhances glucose responsiveness in some ventromedial hypothalamic glucosensing neurons. *Am J Physiol Regul Integr Comp Physiol* 2008;294:R784–R792

123. Osundiji MA, Hurst P, Moore SP, Markkula SP, Yueh CY, Swamy A, Hoashi S, Shaw JS, Riches CH, Heisler LK, Evans ML. Recurrent hypoglycemia increases hypothalamic glucose phosphorylation activity in rats. *Metabolism* 2011;60: 550–556

124. van de Ven KC, Tack CJ, Heerschap A, van der Graaf M, de Galan BE. Patients with type 1 diabetes exhibit altered cerebral metabolism during hypoglycemia. *J Clin Invest* 2013;123:623–629

125. Itoh Y, Esaki T, Shimoji K, Cook M, Law MJ, Kaufman E, Sokoloff L. Dichloroacetate effects on glucose and lactate oxidation by neurons and astroglia in vitro and on glucose utilization by brain in vivo. *Proc Natl Acad Sci USA* 2003;100: 4879–4884

126. Hyder F, Patel AB, Gjedde A, Rothman DL, Behar KL, Shulman RG. Neuronal-glial glucose oxidation and glutaminergic-GABAergic function. *J Cerebr Blood Flow Metab* 2006;26:865–877

127. Mason GF, Petersen KF, Lebon V, Rothman DL, Shulman GI. Increased brain monocarboxylic acid transport and utilization in type 1 diabetes. *Diabetes* 2006;55:929–934

128. Veneman T, Mitrakou A, Mokan M, Cryer P, Gerich J. Effect of hyperketonemia and hyperlacticacidemia on symptoms, cognitive dysfunction, and counterregulatory hormone responses during hypoglycemia in normal humans. *Diabetes* 1994;43:1311–1317

129. Maran A, Cranston I, Lomas J, Macdonald I, Amiel SA. Protection by lactate of cerebral function during hypoglycaemia. *Lancet* 1994;343:16–20

130. Maran A, Crepaldi C, Trupiani S, Lucca T, Jori E, Macdonald IA, Tiengo A, Avogaro A, Del Prato S. Brain function rescue effect of lactate following hypoglycaemia is not an adaptation process in both normal and type I diabetic subjects. *Diabetologia* 2000;43:733–741

131. Wahren J, Ekberg K, Fernqvist-Forbes E, Nair S. Brain substrate utilization during acute hypoglycaemia. *Diabetologia* 1999;42:812–818

132. Lubow JM, Piñón IG, Avogaro A, Cobelli C, Treeson DM, Mandeville KA, Toffolo G, Boyle PJ. Brain oxygen utilization is unchanged by hypoglycemia in normal humans: lactate, alanine, and leucine uptake are not sufficient to offset energy deficit. *Am J Physiol Endocrinol Metab* 2006;290:E149–E153

133. van Hall G, Strømstad M, Rasmussen P, Jans Ø, Zaar M, Gam C, Quistorff B, Secher NH, Nielsen HB. Blood lactate is an important energy source for the human brain. *J Cereb Blood Flow Metab* 2009;29:1121–1129

134. Boumezbeur F, Petersen KF, Cline GW, Mason GF, Behar KL, Shulman GI, Rothman DL. The contribution of blood lactate to brain energy metabolism in humans measured by dynamic ^{13}C nuclear magnetic resonance spectroscopy. *J Neurosci* 2010;30:13983–13991

135. De Feyter HM, Mason GF, Shulman GI, Rothman DL, Petersen KF. Increased brain lactate concentrations without increased lactate oxidation during hypoglycemia in type 1 diabetic individuals. *Diabetes* 2013;62:3075–3080

136. Herzog RI, Jiang L, Herman P, Zhao C, Sanganahalli BG, Mason GF, Hyder F, Rothman DL, Sherwin RS, Behar KL. Lactate preserves neuronal metabolism and function following antecedent recurrent hypoglycemia. *J Clin Invest* 2013;123:1988–1998

137. Chan O, Sherwin R. Influence of VMH fuel sensing on hypoglycemic responses. *Trends Endocrinol Metab* 2013;24:616–624

138. Arbeláez AM, Cryer PE. Lactate and the mechanism of hypoglycemia-associated autonomic failure in diabetes. *Diabetes* 2013;62:3999–4001

139. Terpstra M, Moheet A, Kumar A, Eberly LE, Seaquist E, Öz G. Changes in human brain glutamate concentration during hypoglycemia: insights into cerebral adaptations in hypoglycemia-associated autonomic failure in type 1 diabetes. *J Cereb Blood Flow Metab* 2014;34:876–882

140. Tong Q, Ye CP, McCrimmon RJ, Dhillon H, Choi B, Kramer MD, Yu J, Yang Z, Christiansen LM, Lee CE, Choi CS, Zigman JM, Shulman GI, Sherwin RS, Elmquist JK, Lowell BB. Synaptic glutamate release by ventromedial hypothalamic neurons is part of the neurocircuitry that prevents hypoglycemia. *Cell Metab* 2007;5:383–393

141. Gruetter R. Glycogen: the forgotten cerebral energy store. *J Neurosci Res* 2003; 74:179–183

142. Choi IY, Seaquist ER, Gruetter R. Effect of hypoglycemia on brain glycogen metabolism in vivo. *J Neurosci Res* 2003;72:25–32

143. Herzog RI, Chan O, Yu S, Dziura J, McNay EC, Sherwin RS. Effect of acute and recurrent hypoglycemia on changes in brain glycogen concentration. *Endocrinology* 2008;149:1499–1504

144. Canada SE, Weaver SA, Sharpe SN, Pederson BA. Brain glycogen supercompensation in the mouse after recovery from insulin-induced hypoglycemia. *J Neurosci Res* 2011;89:585–591

145. Öz G, Tesfaye N, Kumar A, Deelchand DK, Eberly LE, Seaquist ER. Brain glycogen content and metabolism in subjects with type 1 diabetes and hypoglycemia unawareness. *J Cereb Blood Flow Metab* 2012;32:256–263

146. Briscoe VJ, Ertl AC, Tate DB, Blair HM, Davis SN. Effects of the selective serotonin reuptake inhibitor, fluoxetine, on counterregulatory responses to hypoglycemia in individuals with T1DM. *Diabetes* 2008;57:3315–3322

147. Briscoe VJ, Ertl AC, Tate DB, Dawling S, Davis SN. Effects of a selective serotonin reuptake inhibitor, fluoxetine, on counterregulatory responses to hypoglycemia in healthy individuals. *Diabetes* 2008;57:2453–2460

148. Sanders NM, Wilkinson CW, Taborsky GJ Jr, Al-Noori S, Daumen W, Zavosh A, Figlewicz DP. The selective serotonin reuptake inhibitor sertraline enhances counterregulatory responses to hypoglycemia. *Am J Physiol Endocrinol Metab* 2008;294:E853–E860

149. Caprio S, Gerety G, Tamborlane WV, Jones T, Diamond M, Jacob R, Sherwin RS. Opiate blockade enhances hypoglycemic counterregulation in normal and insulin-dependent diabetic subjects. *Am J Physiol* 1991;260:E852–E858

150. Vele S, Milman S, Shamoon H, Gabriely I. Opioid receptor blockade improves hypoglycemia-associated autonomic failure in type 1 diabetes mellitus. *J Clin Endocrinol Metab* 2011;96:3424–3431

151. Gabriely, I, Hawkins, M, Vilcu, C, Rossetti, L and Shamoon, H. Fructose amplifies counterregulatory responses to hypoglycemia in humans. *Diabetes* 2002;51:893–900

152. Fan X, Ding Y, Cheng H, Gram DX, Sherwin RS, McCrimmon RJ. Amplified hormonal counterregulatory responses to hypoglycemia in rats after systemic delivery of a SUR-1-selective K(+) channel opener? *Diabetes* 2008;57:3327–3334

153. Cryer PE. Death during intensive glycemic therapy of diabetes: mechanisms and implications. *Am J Med* 2011;124:993–996

154. George PS, Tavendale R, Palmer CNA, McCrimmon RJ. Diazoxide improves hormonal counterregulatory responses to acute hypoglycemia in long-standing type 1 diabetes. *Diabetes* 2015;64:2234–2241

155. Beall C, Haythorne E, Fan X, Du Q, Jovanovic S, Sherwin RS, Ashford ML, McCrimmon RJ. Continuous hypothalamic K_{ATP} activation blunts glucose counter-regulation in vivo in rats and suppresses K_{ATP} conductance in vitro. *Diabetologia* 2013;56:2088–2092

156. Arbeláez AM, Powers WJ, Videen TO, Price JL, Cryer PE. Attenuation of counterregulatory responses to recurrent hypoglycemia by active thalamic inhibition. A mechanism for hypoglycemia-associated autonomic failure. *Diabetes* 2008;57:470–475

157. Arbeláez AM, Rutlin JR, Hershey TG, Powers WJ, Videen TO, Cryer PE. Thalamic activation during slightly subphysiological glycemia in humans. *Diabetes Care* 2012;35:2570–2574

158. Teves D, Videen TO, Cryer PE, Powers WJ. Activation of human medial prefrontal cortex during autonomic responses to hypoglycemia. *Proc Natl Acad Sci USA* 2004;101:6217–6221

159. Teh MM, Dunn JT, Choudhary P, Samarasinghe Y, Macdonald I, O'Doherty M, Marsden P, Reed LJ, Amiel SA. Evolution and resolution of human brain

perfusion responses to the stress of induced hypoglycemia. *NeuroImage* 2010;53: 584–592

160. Bhatnagar S, Viau V, Chu A, Soriano L, Meijer OC, Dallman MF. A cholecystokinin-mediated pathway to the paraventricular thalamus is recruited in chronically stressed rats and regulates hypothalamic-pituitary-adrenal function. *J Neurosci* 2000;20:5564–5573

161. Bhatnagar S, Huber R, Nowak N, Trotter P. Lesions of the posterior paraventricular thalamus block habituation of hypothalamic-pituitary-adrenal responses to repeated restraint. *J Neuroendocrinol* 2002;14:403–410

162. Jaferi A, Nowak N, Bhatnagar S. Negative feedback functions in chronically stressed rats: role of the posterior paraventricular thalamus. *Physiol Behav* 2003;78: 365–373

163. Grissom N, Bhatnagar S. Habituation to repeated stress: get used to it. *Neurobiol Learning Memory* 2009;92:215–224

164. Al-Noori S, Sanders NM, Taborsky GJ Jr, Wilkinson CW, Zavosh A, West C, Sanders CM, Figlewicz DP. Recurrent hypoglycemia alters hypothalamic expression of the regulatory proteins FosB and synaptophysin. *Am J Physiol Regul Integr Comp Physiol* 2008;295:R1446–R1454

165. Konarska M, Stewart RE, McCarty R. Habituation of sympathetic-adrenal medullary responses following exposure to chronic intermittent stress. *Physiol Behav* 1989;45:255–261

166. Konarska M, Stewart RE, McCarty R. Predictability of chronic intermittent stress: effects on sympathetic-adrenal medullary responses of laboratory rats. *Behav Neural Biol* 1990;53:231–243

167. Tesfaye N, Mangia S, De Martino F, Kumar A, Moheet A, Iverson E, Eberly LE, Seaquist ER. Hypoglycemia induced increases in cerebral blood flow are blunted in subjects with type 1 diabetes and hypoglycemia unawareness (abstract). *Diabetes* 2011;60:A79

168. Weinberg MS, Johnson DC, Bhatt AP, Spencer RL. Medial prefrontal cortex activity can disrupt the expression of stress response habituation. *Neuroscience* 2010;168:744–756

169. Cryer PE. Death during intensive glycemic therapy of diabetes: mechanisms and implications. *Am J Med* 2011;124:993–996

170. Deckert T, Poulsen JE, Larsen M. Prognosis of diabetics with diabetes before the age of 31. I. Survival, cause of deaths and complications. *Diabetologia* 1978;14:363–370

171. Tunbridge WMG. Factors contributing to deaths of diabetics under 50 years of age. *Lancet* 1981;2:569–572

172. Laing SP, Swerdlow AJ, Slater SD, Botha JL, Burden AC, Waugh NR, Smith AWM, Hill RD, Bingley PJ, Patterson CC, Qiao Z, Keen H. The British Diabetic Association Cohort Study. I. All-cause mortality in patients with insulin-treated diabetes mellitus. *Diabet Med* 1999;16:459–465

173. Patterson CC, Dahlquist G, Harjutsalo V, Joner G, Feltbower RG, Svensson J, Schober E, Gyürüs E, Castell C, Urbonaité B, Rosenbauer J, Iotova V, Thorsson AV, Soltész G. Early mortality in EURODIAB population-based cohorts of type 1 diabetes diagnosed in childhood since 1989. *Diabetologia* 2007;50:2439–2442

174. Diabetes Control and Complications Trial/Epidemiology of Diabetes Interventions and Complications (DCCT/EDIC) Research Group. Long-term effect of diabetes and its treatment on cognitive function. *N Engl J Med* 2007;356: 1842–1852

175. Diabetes Control and Complications Trial/Epidemiology of Diabetes Interventions and Complications (DCCT/EDIC) Research Group. Association between 7 years of intensive treatment of type 1 diabetes and long-term mortality. *JAMA* 2015;313:45–53

176. Feltbower RG, Bodansky HJ, Patterson CC, Parslow RC, Stephenson CR, Reynolds C, McKinney PA. Acute complications and drug misuse are important causes of death for children and young adults with type 1 diabetes. *Diabetes Care* 2008;31:922–926

177. Skrivarhaug T, Bangstad H-J, Stene LC, Sandvik L, Hanssen KF, Joner G. Long-term mortality in a nationwide cohort of childhood-onset type 1 diabetic patients in Norway. *Diabetologia* 2006;49:298–305

178. Gerich JE. Oral hypoglycemic agents. *N Engl J Med* 1989;321:1231–1245

179. Holstein A, Egberts EH. Risk of hypoglycaemia with oral antidiabetic agents in patients with type 2 diabetes. *Exp Clin Endocrinol Metab* 2003;111:405–414

180. Bonds DE, Miller ME, Bergenstal RM, Buse JB, Byington RP, Cutler JA, Dudl RJ, Ismail-Beigi F, Kimel AR, Hoogwerf B, Horowitz KR, Savage PJ, Seaquist ER, Simmons DL, Sivitz WI, Speril-Hillen JM, Sweeney ME. The association between symptomatic, severe hypoglycaemia and mortality in type 2 diabetes: retrospective epidemiological analysis of the ACCORD study. *BMJ* 2010;340:b4909

181. Auer RN. Progress review: hypoglycemic brain damage. *Stroke* 1986;17:699–708

182. Suh SW, Hamby AM, Swanson RA. Hypoglycemia, brain energetic and hypoglycemic neuronal death. *GLIA* 2007;55:1280–1286

183. Cryer PE. Hypoglycemia, functional brain failure, and brain death. *J Clin Invest* 2007;117:868–870

184. Witsch J, Neugebauer H, Flechsenhar J, Jüttler E. Hypoglycemic encephalopathy: a case series and literature review on outcome determination. *J Neurol* 2012; 259:2172–2181

185. Ikeda T, Takahashi T, Sato A, Tanaka H, Igarashi S, Fujita N, Kuwabara T, Kanazawa M, Nishizawa M, Shimohata T. Predictors of outcome in hypoglycemic encephalopathy. *Diabetes Res Clin Pract* 2013;101:159–163

186. Suh SW, Aoyama K, Chen Y, Garnier P, Matsumori Y, Gum E, Liu J, Swanson RA. Hypoglycemic neuronal death and cognitive impairment are prevented by poly(ADP-ribose) polymerase inhibitors administered after hypoglycemia. *J Neurosci* 2003;23:10681–10690

187. Suh SW, Gum ET, Hamby AM, Chan PH, Swanson RA. Hypoglycemic neuronal death is triggered by glucose reperfusion and activation of neuronal NADPH oxidase. *J Clin Invest* 2007;117:910–918

188. Stahn A, Pistrosch F, Ganz X, Teige M, Koehler C, Bornstein S, Hanefeld M. Relationship between hypoglycemic episodes and ventricular arrhythmias in patients with type 2 diabetes and cardiovascular diseases: silent hypoglycemias and silent arrhythmias. *Diabetes Care* 2014;37:516–520

189. Chow E, Bernjak A, Williams S, Fawdry RA, Hibbert S, Freeman J, Sheridan PJ, Heller SR. Risk of cardiac arrhythmias during hypoglycemia in patients with type 2 diabetes and cardiovascular risk. *Diabetes* 2014;63:1738–1747

190. Lee SP, Yeoh L, Harris ND, Davies CM, Robinson RT, Leathard A, Newman C, Macdonald IA, Heller SR. Influence of autonomic neuropathy on QTc interval lengthening during hypoglycemia in type 1 diabetes. *Diabetes* 2004;53:1535–1542

191. Laitinen T, Lyyra-Laitinen T, Huopio H, Vauhkonen I, Halonen T, Hartikainen J, Niskanen L, Laakso M. Electrocardiographic alterations during hyperinsulinemic hypoglycemia in healthy subjects. *Ann Noninvasive Electrocardiol* 2008; 13:97–105

192. Osadchii OE. Mechanisms of hypokalemia-induced ventricular arrhythmogenicity. *Fundam Clin Pharmacol* 2010;24:547–559

193. Nordin C. The case for hypoglycaemia as a proarrhythmic event: basic and clinical evidence. *Diabetologia* 2010;53:1552–1561

194. Nordin C. The proarrhythmic effect of hypoglycemia: evidence for increased risk from ischemia and bradycardia. *Acta Diabetol* 2014;51:5–14

195. Frier BM, Schernthaner G, Heller SR. Hypoglycemia and cardiovascular risks. *Diabetes Care* 2011;34(Suppl. 2):S132–S137

196. Chow E, Heller SR. Pathophysiology of the effects of hypoglycemia on the cardiovascular system. *Diabetic Hypogly* 2012;5:3–8

197. Haugaa KH, Bos JM, Tarrell RF, Morlan BW, Caraballo PJ, Ackerman MJ. Institution-wide QT alert system identifies patients with a high risk of mortality. *Mayo Clin Proc* 2013;88:315–325

198. Cox AJ, Azeem A, Yeboah J, Soliman EZ, Aggarwal SR, Bertoni AG, Carr JJ, Freedman BI, Herrington DM, Bowden DW. Heart rate-corrected QT interval is an independent predictor of all-cause and cardiovascular mortality in individuals with type 2 diabetes: The Diabetes Heart Study. *Diabetes Care* 2014;37: 1454–1461

199. Lee S, Harris ND, Robinson RT, Yeoh L, Macdonald IA, Heller SR. Effects of adrenaline and potassium on QTc interval and QT dispersion in man. *Eur J Clin Invest* 2003;33:93–98

200. Robinson RT, Harris ND, Ireland RH, Lee S, Newman C, Heller SR. Mechanisms of abnormal cardiac repolarization during insulin-induced hypoglycemia. *Diabetes* 2003;52:1469–1474

201. Lee SP, Harris ND, Robinson RT, Davies C, Ireland R, Macdonald IA, Heller SR. Effect of atenolol on QTc interval lengthening during hypoglycaemia in type 1 diabetes. *Diabetologia* 2005;48:1269–1272

202. Gill GV, Woodward A, Casson IF, Weston PJ. Cardiac arrhythmia and nocturnal hypoglycaemia in type 1 diabetes— the "dead in bed" syndrome revisited. *Diabetologia* 2009;52:42–45

203. Murphy NP, Ford-Adams ME, Ong KK, Harris ND, Keane SM, Davies C, Ireland RH, Macdonald IA, Knight EJ, Edge JA, Heller SR, Dunger DB. Prolonged cardiac repolarisation during spontaneous nocturnal hypoglycaemia in children and adolescents with type 1 diabetes. *Diabetologia* 2004;47:1940–1947

204. Robinson RT, Harris ND, Ireland RH, Macdonald IA, Heller SR. Changes in cardiac repolarization during clinical episodes of nocturnal hypoglycaemia in adults with type 1 diabetes. *Diabetologia* 2004;47:312–315

205. Tsujimoto T, Yamamoto-Honda R, Kajio H, Kishimoto M, Noto H, Hachiya R, Kimura A, Kakei M, Noda M. Vital signs, QT prolongation, and newly diagnosed cardiovascular disease during severe hypoglycemia in type 1 and type 2 diabetic patients. *Diabetes Care* 2014;37:217–225

206. Beom JW, Kim JM, Chung EJ, Kim JY, Ko SY, Na SD, Kim CH, Park G, Kang MY. Corrected QT interval prolongation during severe hypoglycemia without hypokalemia in patients with type 2 diabetes. *Diabetes Metab J* 2013;37:190–195

207. Tsujimoto T, Yamamoto-Honda R, Kajio H, Kishimoto M, Noto H, Hachiya R, Kimura A, Kakei M, Noda M. Vital signs, QT prolongation, and newly diagnosed cardiovascular disease during severe hypoglycemia in type 1 and type 2 diabetic patients. *Diabetes Care* 2014;37:217–225

208. Pistrosch F, Ganz X, Bornstein SR, Birkenfeld AL, Henkel E, Hanefeld M. Risk of and risk factors for hypoglycemia and associated arrhythmias in patients with type 2 diabetes and cardiovascular disease: a cohort study under real-world conditions. *Acta Diabetol* 2015. doi:10.1007/s00592-015-0727-2

209. Caduff A, Lutz HU, Heinemann L, Di Benedetto G, Talary MS, Theander S. Dynamics of blood electrolytes in repeated hyper- and/or hypoglycaemic events in patients with type 1 diabetes. *Diabetologia* 2011;54:2678–2689

210. Reno CM, Daphna-Iken D, Chen YS, VanderWeele J, Jethi K, Fisher SJ. Severe hypoglycemia-induced lethal cardiac arrhythmias are mediated by sympathoadrenal activation. *Diabetes* 2013;62:3570–3581

211. ORIGIN Trial Investigators. Does hypoglycemia increase the risk of cardiovascular events? A report from the ORIGIN trial. *Eur Heart J* 2013;34:3137–3144

212. VanderWeele JJ, Daphna-Iken D, Chen YS, Hoffman RS, Clark AL, Fisher SJ. Antecedent recurrent hypoglycemia reduces lethal cardiac arrhythmias induced by severe hypoglycemia in diabetic rats (abstract). *Diabetes* 2014;63(Suppl. 1):39

213. Zoungas S, Patel A, Chalmers J, de Galan BE, Li Q, Billot L, Woodward M, Nimomiya T, Neal B, MacMahon S, Grobbee DE, Kengne AP, Marre M, Heller S and the ADVANCE Collaborative Group. Severe hypoglycemia and risks of vascular events and death. *N Engl J Med* 2010;363:1410–1418

214. Seaquist ER, Miller ME, Bonds DE, Feinglos M, Goff DC Jr, Peterson K, Senior P, for the ACCORD Investigators. The impact of frequent and unrecognized hypoglycaemia on mortality in the ACCORD study. *Diabetes Care* 2012;35:409–414

215. Cryer PE. Hypoglycemia-associated autonomic failure in diabetes: maladaptive, adaptive, or both? *Diabetes* 2015;64:2322–2323

4
Risk Factors for Hypoglycemia in Diabetes

The risk factors for hypoglycemia in people with diabetes (see Table 4.1)[1–6] follow directly from the pathophysiology of glucose counterregulation in diabetes (see Chapter 3). The principle is that iatrogenic hypoglycemia in type 1 diabetes (T1D) and advanced type 2 diabetes (T2D) is typically the result of the interplay of relative or absolute therapeutic insulin excess and compromised physiological and behavioral defenses against falling plasma glucose concentrations—that is, hypoglycemia-associated autonomic failure (HAAF) in diabetes.

People with diabetes are not immune to hypoglycemia caused by mechanisms other than the treatment of their diabetes.[7] Those include *1*) an array of drugs,[8,9] including alcohol; *2*) critical illnesses such as renal, hepatic, or cardiac failure, sepsis, or inanition; *3*) hormone deficiency states, such as adrenocortical failure; *4*) nonislet tumor hypoglycemia; *5*) endogenous hyperinsulinism; and *6*) accidental, surreptitious, or even malicious hypoglycemia. Aside from drug effects, those mechanisms are uncommon.

Relative or Absolute Insulin Excess

The conventional risk factors for hypoglycemia in diabetes[1–6] are based on the premise that relative or absolute therapeutic insulin excess is the sole determinant of risk. That excess may be either endogenous (sulfonylurea, or

DOI: 10.2337/9781580406499.04

glinide, stimulated) or exogenous insulin. People with T2D using a sulfonylurea or a glinide and people with T1D or T2D using insulin are at ongoing risk for episodes of hyperinsulinemia because of the pharmacodynamic and pharmacokinetic imperfections of those therapies. Sulfonylureas stimulate insulin secretion even at normal (or low) plasma glucose concentrations,[10] and the circulating levels of injected insulin do not decrease as plasma glucose concentrations decline. Indeed, therapeutic hyperinsulinemia is a prerequisite for the development of hypoglycemia in diabetes (see Chapter 3). Whereas those episodes can include absolute hyperinsulinemia, the conventional risk factors also focus on relative hyperinsulinemia—that is, insulin levels insufficient to cause hypoglycemia under most conditions but high enough to cause hypoglycemia in the setting of decreased exogenous glucose delivery or endogenous glucose production, increased glucose utilization, or increased sensitivity to insulin (see Table 4.1).

Absolute or relative therapeutic insulin excess occurs when sulfonylurea, glinide, or insulin doses are excessive, ill-timed, or of the wrong type. Relative insulin excess occurs under a variety of conditions. It occurs when exogenous glucose delivery is decreased, as it is after missed (or low-carbohydrate) meals and during the overnight fast; when endogenous glucose production is decreased, as it is after alcohol ingestion; when glucose utilization is increased, as it is during or shortly after exercise; and when sensitivity to insulin

Table 4.1—Risk Factors for Hypoglycemia in Diabetes

Relative or absolute insulin excess:
1. Insulin or insulin secretagogue doses are excessive, ill-timed, or of the wrong type.
2. Exogenous glucose delivery is decreased (e.g., after missed meals and during the overnight fast).
3. Endogenous glucose production is decreased (e.g., after alcohol ingestion).
4. Glucose utilization is increased (e.g., during and shortly after exercise).
5. Sensitivity to insulin is increased (e.g., after weight loss or improved glycemic control and in the middle of the night).
6. Insulin clearance is decreased (e.g., with renal failure).
Hypoglycemia-associated autonomic failure (defective glucose counterregulation and hypoglycemia unawareness):
1. Absolute endogenous insulin deficiency
2. A history of severe hypoglycemia, hypoglycemia unawareness, or both as well as recent antecedent hypoglycemia, prior exercise, and sleep
3. Aggressive glycemic therapy per se (lower A1C levels, lower glycemic goals, or both)

is increased, in the long term after weight loss or improved glycemic control and in the short term in the middle of the night. Renal failure increases the risk of iatrogenic hypoglycemia in diabetes in part because *1*) the kidneys are normally the site of ~40% of the clearance of insulin from the circulation and reduced renal function reduces the clearance of insulin,[11] resulting in the need for a progressive decrease in insulin dosing to avoid hypoglycemia,[12] and *2*) the kidneys are normally the site of about 25% of endogenous glucose production[13,14] that is stimulated by epinephrine,[13] increases during hypoglycemia,[14] and likely decreases as renal function declines. Additional factors could include decreased metabolism of sulfonylureas and malnutrition, resulting in hepatic glycogen depletion and decreased mobilization of gluconeogenic precursors from muscle and fat. Alcohol causes hypoglycemia by inhibiting gluconeogenesis.[7] Consumption of alcohol in the evening has been shown to cause hypoglycemia the following morning in patients with T1D.[15]

People with diabetes and their caregivers deal with these risk factors whenever hypoglycemia becomes a problem. Clearly, in a given patient, each of these needs to be considered carefully and the regimen should be adjusted appropriately. Nonetheless, aside from the first risk factor, these other factors explain only a minority of episodes of hypoglycemia.[16] In most instances, other risk factors, specifically those indicative of HAAF, determine whether a given episode of therapeutic hyperinsulinemia does, or does not, result in an episode of hypoglycemia (see Chapter 3).

Hypoglycemia-Associated Autonomic Failure

The risk factors for hypoglycemia indicative of HAAF (see Table 4.1)[1–6] include the degree of absolute endogenous insulin deficiency[17–23]; a history of severe hypoglycemia, hypoglycemia unawareness, or both[18–20,24] and conditions known to cause HAAF (recent antecedent hypoglycemia, prior exercise, or sleep); and aggressive glycemic therapy per se.[5,18–21,24–26]

As discussed earlier, defective glucose counterregulation, one of the components of HAAF, develops in the setting of absent decrements in insulin and absent increments in glucagon, and both of these pathophysiological features stem fundamentally from β-cell failure (see Chapter 3).[27] Thus, the degree of absolute endogenous insulin deficiency determines both the extent to which insulin levels will not decrease and the extent to which glucagon levels will not increase as plasma glucose concentrations fall in response to therapeutic hyperinsulinemia. Longer duration of diabetes is associated with the loss of endogenous insulin secretion, early in T1D and later in T2D. The extent to which age per se (as compared with the duration of diabetes and progressive deterioration of β-cell function) plays a role is unclear, but rather subtle abnormalities of glucose counterregulatory defenses have been reported in older people.[28,29] Thus, longer duration of diabetes is associated with a higher frequency of severe hypoglycemia[22,30] probably because of further decreased insulin secretion. Indeed, there is evidence of lower rates of severe hypoglycemia in patients who have some degree of residual insulin secretion.[21,31,32]

A history of severe hypoglycemia indicates, and a history of hypoglycemia unawareness implies, recent antecedent hypoglycemia. As discussed in Chapter 3,[27] recent antecedent hypoglycemia causes an attenuated sympathoadrenal response to subsequent hypoglycemia, the key feature of defective glucose counterregulation and the cause of hypoglycemia unawareness, which are the two components of HAAF, and thus the pathogenesis of iatrogenic hypoglycemia. In addition to recent antecedent hypoglycemia, prior exercise and sleep cause HAAF.

As documented in clinical trials with sample sizes large enough to demonstrate beneficial effects in T1D[33,34] and T2D,[24,35–37] and confirmed in a meta-analysis that included 12 smaller trials in T1D,[38] if all other factors are the same, patients treated to lower, compared with higher, A1C levels are at higher risk for hypoglycemia.[5] Stated differently, studies with a control group treated to a higher A1C level consistently report higher rates of hypoglycemia in the group treated to a lower A1C level in T1D[33,34,38] and T2D.[24,35–37] Thus, although iatrogenic hypoglycemia can occur in those with relatively high A1C values and observational data suggest a less marked relationship,[39,40] a relationship between lower A1C levels and higher rates of hypoglycemia continues to be observed.[41,42] A lower A1C is a risk factor for hypoglycemia. Indeed, lower mean plasma glucose concentrations and greater plasma glucose variability are also associated with a higher risk of hypoglycemia.[43] That does not mean, of course, that one cannot both improve glycemic control and minimize the risk for hypoglycemia in individual patients (Chapter 6).[1–4,44–48]

These risk factors for HAAF also apply to young children with T1D.[49,50] Improved glycemic control before and during pregnancy is particularly important in the short term because it improves pregnancy outcomes in women with T1D. But, it increases the frequency of hypoglycemia substantially.[51–54] In one series, 45% of 108 women with T1D suffered severe hypoglycemia during their pregnancies; compared with a prepregnancy rate of 110 per 100 patient-years, the incidence was the equivalent of 530, 240, and 50 episodes per 100 patient-years in the first, second, and third trimesters, respectively.[52] The risk factors for HAAF—previous severe hypoglycemia,[51,52] impaired awareness of hypoglycemia,[52] and lower A1C levels[51]—also are associated with higher rates of severe hypoglycemia in pregnant women with T1D.

A relationship between the deletion (D) allele of the angiotensin-converting enzyme (ACE) gene and its associated higher serum ACE activity and severe hypoglycemia has been reported in some,[55–57] but not all,[58,59] studies in T1D. It also has been reported in some[60] but not all[61] studies in T2D with a weak relationship in another study in T2D.[62] The mechanism of this apparent association is unclear. It has been noted that healthy individuals[63] and patients with T1D[64] with higher serum ACE activities are more susceptible to cognitive dysfunction during hypoglycemia, a plausible factor in the pathogenesis of severe hypoglycemia. In one contrast of nine patients with T1D and high renin-angiotensin system (RAS) activity and nine patients with low RAS activity, the high RAS group had reduced symptoms of hypoglycemia, had a tenfold higher incidence of prior severe hypoglycemia, and tended to have lower glucagon and epinephrine responses to hypoglycemia.[64] Thus, it is conceivable that conventional mechanisms (i.e., HAAF) explain the high frequency of severe hypoglycemia and that the higher serum ACE activity might be a result rather than the cause of hypoglycemia. That result, however, would not explain the association of severe hypoglycemia with the DD genotype observed in some studies.[55,60]

References

1. Cryer PE, Davis SN, Shamoon H. Hypoglycemia in diabetes. *Diabetes Care* 2003;26:1902–1912

2. Cryer PE. Diverse causes of hypoglycemia-associated autonomic failure in diabetes. *N Engl J Med* 2004;350:2272–2279

3. Cryer PE. The barrier of hypoglycemia in diabetes. *Diabetes* 2008;57:3169–3176

4. Cryer PE. Hypoglycemia in diabetes. In *Textbook of Diabetes.* 4th ed. Holt RIG, Cockram C, Flyvbjerg A, Goldstein BJ, Eds. Oxford, U.K., Wiley-Blackwell, 2010, p. 528–545

5. Cryer PE. Glycemic goals in diabetes: trade-off between glycemic control and iatrogenic hypoglycemia. *Diabetes* 2014;63:2188–2195

6. Cryer PE. Hypoglycemia. In *Williams Textbook of Endocrinology*. 13th ed. Melmed S, Polonsky KS, Larsen PR, Kronenberg HM, Eds. Philadelphia, Elsevier, 2016, p. 1582–1607

7. Cryer PE, Axelrod L, Grossman AB, Heller SR, Montori VM, Seaquist ER, Service FJ. Evaluation and management of adult hypoglycemic disorders. *J Clin Endocrinol Metab* 2009;94:709–728

8. Murad MH, Coto-Yglesias F, Wang AT, Sheidaee N, Mullan RJ, Elamin MB, Erwin PJ, Montori VM. Drug-induced hypoglycemia: a systemic review. *J Clin Endocrinol Metab* 2009;94:741–745

9. Ben Salem C, Fathallah N, Hmouda H, Bouraoui K. Drug-induced hypoglycaemia: an update. *Drug Saf* 2011;34:21–45

10. Riefflin A, Ayyagari U, Manley SE, Holman RR, Levy JC. The effect of glibenclamide on insulin secretion at normal glucose concentrations. *Diabetologia* 2015;58:43–49

11. Rabkin R, Simon NM, Steiner S, Colwell JA. Effect of renal disease on renal uptake and excretion of insulin in man. *N Engl J Med* 1970;282:182–187

12. Biesenbach G, Raml A, Schmekal B, Eichbauer-Sturm G. Decreased insulin requirement in relation to GFR in nephropathic type 1 and insulin-treated type 2 diabetic patients. *Diabet Med* 2003;20:642–645

13. Stumvoll M, Chintalapudi U, Perriello G, Welle S, Gutierrez O, Gerich J. Uptake and release of glucose by the human kidney. Postabsorptive rates and responses to epinephrine. *J Clin Invest* 1995;96:2528–2533

14. Cersosimo E, Garlick P, Ferretti J. Renal glucose production during insulin-induced hypoglycemia in humans. *Diabetes* 1999;48:261–266

15. Turner BC, Jenkins E, Kerr D, Sherwin RS, Cavan DA. The effect of evening alcohol consumption on next-morning glucose control in type 1 diabetes. *Diabetes Care* 2001;24:1888–1893

16. Diabetes Control and Complications Trial Research Group (DCCT). Epidemiology of severe hypoglycemia in the Diabetes Control and Complications Trial. *Am J Med* 1991;90:450–459

17. Fukuda M, Tanaka A, Tahara Y, Ikegami H, Yamamoto Y, Kumahara Y, Shima K. Correlation between minimal secretory capacity of pancreatic β-cells and stability of diabetic control. *Diabetes* 1988;37:81–88

18. Diabetes Control and Complications Trial Research Group (DCCT). Hypoglycemia in the Diabetes Control and Complications Trial. *Diabetes* 1997;46: 271–286

19. Mühlhauser I, Overmann H, Bender R, Bott U, Berger M. Risk factors for severe hypoglycaemia in adult patients with type 1 diabetes—a prospective population based study. *Diabetologia* 1997;41:1274–1282

20. Allen C, LeCaire T, Palta M, Daniels K, Meredith M, D'Alessio DJ, for the Wisconsin Diabetes Registry Project. Risk factors for frequent and severe hypoglycemia in type 1 diabetes. *Diabetes Care* 2001;24:1878–1881

21. Steffes MW, Sibley S, Jackson M, Thomas W. β-cell function and the development of diabetes related complications in the Diabetes Control and Complications Trial. *Diabetes Care* 2003;26:832–836

22. U.K. Hypoglycaemia Study Group (UK Hypo Group). Risk of hypoglycaemia in types 1 and 2 diabetes: effects of treatment modalities and their duration. *Diabetologia* 2007;50:1140–1147

23. Chow LS, Chen H, Miller MS, Marcovina SM, Seaquist SR. Biomarkers related to severe hypoglycaemia and lack of good glycaemic control in ACCORD. *Diabetologia* 2015;58:1160–1166

24. Wright AD, Cull CA, MacLeod KM, Holman RR, for the UKPDS Group. Hypoglycemia in type 2 diabetic patients randomized to and maintained on monotherapy with diet, sulfonylurea, metformin, or insulin for 6 years from diagnosis: UKPDS 73. *J Diabetes Complications* 2006;20:395–401

25. Lüddeke H-J, Sreenan S, Aczel S, Maxeiner S, Yeniqun M, Kozlovski P, Gydesen H, Dornhorst A, on behalf of the PREDICTIVE Study Group. PREDICTIVE—A global, prospective observational study to evaluate insulin detemir treatment in types 1 and 2 diabetes: baseline characteristics and predictors of hypoglycemia from the European cohort. *Diabetes Obes Metab* 2007;9:428–434

26. Hemmingsen B, Lund SS, Gluud C, Vaag A, Almdal TP, Hemmingsen C, Wetterslev J. Targeting intensive glycaemic control versus targeting conventional glycaemic control for type 2 diabetes mellitus. *Cochrane Database Syst Rev* 2013;11:CD008143. doi:10.1002/14651858.CD008143.pub3

27. Cryer PE. Mechanisms of hypoglycemia-associated autonomic failure in diabetes. *N Engl J Med* 2013;369:362–372

28. Marker JC, Cryer PE, Clutter WE. Attenuated glucose recovery from hypoglycemia in the elderly. *Diabetes* 1992;41:671–678

29. Meneilly GS, Cheung E, Tuokko H. Altered responses to hypoglycemia of healthy elderly people. *J Clin Endocrinol Metab* 1994;78:1341–1348

30. Weinstock RS, Xing D, Maahs DM, Michels A, Rickels MR, Peters AL, Bergenstal RM, Harris B, Dubose SN, Miller KM, Beck RW, Network TDEC. Severe hypoglycemia and diabetic ketoacidosis in adults with type 1 diabetes: results from the T1D Exchange Clinic Registry. *J Clin Endocrinol Metab* 2013;98:3411–3419

31. Sorensen JS, Johannesen J, Pociot F, Kristensen K, Thomsen J, Hertel NT, Kjaersgaard P, Brorsson C, Birkebaek NH, Danish Society for Diabetes in Childhood and Adolescence. Residual β-Cell function 3-6 years after onset of type 1 diabetes reduces risk of severe hypoglycemia in children and adolescents. *Diabetes Care* 2013;36:3454–3459

32. Lachin JM, McGee P, Palmer JP, Group DER. Impact of C-peptide preservation on metabolic and clinical outcomes in the Diabetes Control and Complications Trial. *Diabetes* 2014;63:739–748

33. Diabetes Control and Complications Trial Research Group (DCCT). The effect of intensive treatment of diabetes on the development and progression of long-term complications in insulin dependent diabetes mellitus. *N Engl J Med* 1993;329:977–986

34. Reichard P, Pihl M. Mortality and treatment side-effects during long-term intensified conventional insulin treatment in the Stockholm Diabetes Intervention Study. *Diabetes* 1994;43:313–317

35. ADVANCE Collaborative Group (ADVANCE). Intensive blood glucose control and vascular outcomes in patients with type 2 diabetes. *N Engl J Med* 2008;358:2560–2572

36. Action to Control Cardiovascular Risk in Diabetes Study Group (ACCORD). Effects of intensive glucose lowering in type 2 diabetes. *N Engl J Med* 2008;358:2545–2559

37. Duckworth W, Abraira C, Moritz T, Reda D, Emanuele N, Reaven PD, et al. for the Veterans Affairs Diabetes Therapy (VADT) Investigators. Glucose control and vascular complications in veterans with type 2 diabetes. *N Engl J Med* 2009;360:129–139

38. Egger M, Davey Smith G, Stettler C, Diem P. Risk of adverse effects of intensified treatment in insulin-dependent diabetes mellitus: a meta-analysis. *Diabet Med* 1997;14:919–928

39. Cooper MN, O'Connell SM, Davis EA, Jones TW. A population-based study of risk factors for severe hypoglycaemia in a contemporary cohort of childhood-onset type 1 diabetes. *Diabetologia* 2013;56:2164–2170

40. Johnson SR, Cooper MN, Jones TW, Davis SA. Long-term outcome of insulin pump therapy in children with type 1 diabetes assessed in a large population-based case-control study. *Diabetologia* 2013;56:2392–2400

41. Lipska KJ, Warton EM, Huang ES, Moffet HH, Inzucchi SE, Krumholz HM, Karter AJ. HbA_{1c} and risk of severe hypoglycemia in type 2 diabetes: the Diabetes and Aging Study. *Diabetes Care* 2013;36:3535–3542

42. Monami M, Dicembrini I, Kundisova L, Zannoni S, Nreru B, Mannucci E. A meta-analysis of the hypoglycemic risk in randomized controlled trials with sulfonylurea in patients with type 2 diabetes. *Diabetes Obes Metab* 2014;16: 833–840

43. Kilpatrick ES, Rigby AS, Goode K, Atkin SL. Relating mean blood glucose and glucose variability to the risk of multiple episodes of hypoglycaemia in type 1 diabetes. *Diabetologia* 2007;50:2553–2561

44. Cryer PE. Elimination of hypoglycemia from the lives of people with diabetes. *Diabetes* 2011;60:24–27

45. Rossetti P, Porcellati F, Bolli GB, Fanelli CG. Prevention of hypoglycemia while achieving good glycemic control in type 1 diabetes. Diabetes Care 2008;31(Supp.l 2):S113–S120

46. Hopkins D, Lawrence I, Mansell P, Thompson G, Amiel S, Campbell M, Heller S. Improved biomedical and psychological outcomes 1 year after structured education in flexible insulin therapy for people with type 1 diabetes: the U.K. DAFNE experience. *Diabetes Care* 2012;35:1638–1642

47. Little SA, Leelarathna L, Walkinshaw E, Tan HK, Chapple O, Lubina-Solomon A, Chadwick TJ, Barendse S, Stocken DD, Brennand C, Marshall SM, Wood R, Speight J, Kerr D, Flanagan D, Heller SR, Evans ML, Shaw JAM. Recovery of hypoglycemia awareness in long-standing type 1 diabetes: a multicenter 2 × 2 factorial randomized controlled trial comparing insulin pump with multiple daily injections and continuous with conventional glucose self-monitoring (HypoCOMPaSS). *Diabetes Care* 2014;37:2114–2122

48. International Hypoglycaemia Study Group. Minimizing hypoglycemia in diabetes. *Diabetes Care* 2015;38:1583–1591

49. Brambilla P, Bougneres PF, Santiago JV, Chaussain JL, Pouplard A, Castano L. Glucose counterregulation in pre-school-age diabetic children with recurrent hypoglycemia during conventional treatment. *Diabetes* 1987;36:300–304

50. Jones TW, Boulware SD, Kraemer DT, Caprio S, Sherwin RS, Tamborlane WV. Independent effects of youth and poor diabetes control on responses to hypoglycemia in children. *Diabetes* 1991;40:358–363

51. Evers IM, ter Braak EWMT, de Valk HW, van der Schoot B, Janssen N, Visser GHA. Risk indicators predictive of severe hypoglycemia during the first trimester of type 1 diabetic pregnancy. *Diabetes Care* 2002;25:554–559

52. Nielsen LR, Pedersen-Bjergaard U, Thorsteinsson B, Johansen M, Damm P, Mathiesen ER. Hypoglycemia in pregnant women with type 1 diabetes. *Diabetes Care* 2008;31:9–14

53. Robertson H, Pearson DWM, Gold AE. Severe hypoglycaemia during pregnancy in women with type 1 diabetes is common and planning pregnancy does not decrease the risk. *Diabet Med* 2009;26:824–826

54. Heller S, Damm P, Mersebach H, Skjøth TV, Kaaja R, Hod M, Durán-Garcia, McCance D, Mathiesen ER. Hypoglycemia in type 1 diabetic pregnancy. *Diabetes Care* 2010;33:473–477

55. Pedersen-Bjergaard U, Agerholm-Larsen B, Pramming S, Hougaard P, Thorsteinsson B. Activity of angiotensin-converting enzyme and risk of severe hypoglycemia in type 1 diabetes mellitus. *Lancet* 2001;357:1248–1253

56. Nordfeldt S, Samuelsson U. Serum ACE predicts severe hypoglycemia in children and adolescents with type 1 diabetes. *Diabetes Care* 2003;26:274–278

57. Pedersen-Bjergaard U, Nielsen SL, Akram K, Perrild H, Nordestgaard BG, Montgomery HE, Pramming S, Thorsteinsson B. Angiotensin converting enzyme and angiotensin II receptor subtype 2 genotypes in type 1 diabetes and severe hypoglycaemia requiring emergency treatment: a case cohort study. *Pharmacogenet Genomics* 2009;19:864–868

58. Bulsara MK, Holman CDJ, van Bockxmeer FM, Davis EA, Gallego PH, Beilby JP, Palmer LJ, Choong C, Jones TW. The relationship between ACE genotype and risk of severe hypoglycaemia in a large population-based cohort of children and adolescents with type 1 diabetes. *Diabetologia* 2007;50:965–971

59. Johannesen J, Svensson J, Bergholdt R, Eising S, Gramstrup H, Frandsen E, Dick-Nielsen J, Hansen L, Pociot F, Mortensen HB, the Danish Society for Diabetes in Childhood and Adolescence. Hypoglycemia, S-ACE and ACE genotypes in a

Danish nationwide population of children and adolescents with type 1 diabetes. *Pediatr Diabetes* 2010;12:100–106

60. Davis WA, Brown SGA, Jacobs IG, Bulsara M, Beilby J, Bruce DG, Davis TME. Angiotensin converting enzyme insertion/deletion polymorphism and severe hypoglycemia complicating type 2 diabetes: the Fremantle Diabetes Study. *J Clin Endocrinol Metab* 2011;96:E696–E700

61. Freathy RM, Lonnen KF, Steele AM, Minton JAL, Frayling TM, Hattersley AT, MacLeod KM. The impact of the angiotensin-converting enzyme insertion/deletion polymorphism on severe hypoglycemia in type 2 diabetes. *Rev Diabet Stud* 2006;3:76–81

62. Zammitt N, Geddes J, Warren RE, Marioni R, Ashby PJ, Frier BM. Serum angiotensin-converting enzyme and frequency of severe hypoglycaemia in type 1 diabetes: does a relationship exist? *Diabet Med* 2007;24:1449–1454

63. Pedersen-Bjergaard U, Thomsen CE, Høgenhaven H, Smed A, Kjær TW, Holst JJ, Dela F, Hilsted L, Frandsen E, Pramming S, Thorsteinsson B. Angiotensin-converting enzyme activity and cognitive impairment during hypoglycaemia in healthy humans. *JRAAS* 2008;9:37–48

64. Høi-Hansen T, Pedersen-Bjergaard U, Andersen RD, Kristensen PL, Thomsen C, Kjær T, Høgenhaven H, Smed A, Holst JJ, Dela F, Boomsma F, Thorsteinsson B. Cognitive performance, symptoms and counter-regulation during hypoglycaemia in patients with type 1 diabetes and high or low renin-angiotensin system activity. *J Renin Angiotensin Aldosterone Syst* 2009;10:216–229

5
The Clinical Definition and Classification of Hypoglycemia in Diabetes

The Glucose Alert Value

The American Diabetes Association (ADA) Workgroup on Hypoglycemia[1] and the ADA/Endocrine Society Workgroup on Hypoglycemia[2] defined hypoglycemia in diabetes as "all episodes of abnormally low plasma glucose concentration that expose the individual to potential harm." That includes asymptomatic hypoglycemia because that also impairs defense against subsequent hypoglycemia (Chapter 3).[3–5] Because the glycemic threshold for symptoms, among other responses to hypoglycemia, shifts to lower plasma glucose concentrations in patients with recurrent hypoglycemia and to higher plasma glucose concentrations in those with poorly controlled diabetes,[6–8] it is not possible to state a single plasma glucose concentration that defines hypoglycemia. Nonetheless, the ADA Workgroup,[1] the ADA/Endocrine Society Workgroup,[2] and the International Hypoglyceamia Study Group[9] recommended that people with drug-treated diabetes (implicitly those treated with a sulfonylurea, a glinide, or insulin) become concerned about developing hypoglycemia at a self-monitored plasma glucose concentration of ≤70 mg/dL (≤3.9 mmol/L). Within the error of self–plasma glucose monitoring (or continuous glucose monitoring) devices, that glucose level approximates the lower limit of the nondiabetic postabsorptive plasma glucose concentration

DOI: 10.2337/9781580406499.05

range and the normal glycemic thresholds for activation of physiological glucose counterregulatory systems (see Chapter 2),[10] and the level is low enough to reduce glycemic defenses against subsequent hypoglycemia,[5] in individuals without diabetes. Indeed, impaired performance of a critical task, driving, has been documented at plasma glucose concentrations in the 61–70 mg/dL (3.4–4.0 mmol/L) range in patients with type 1 diabetes (T1D).[11] That glucose level is higher than the plasma glucose levels required to produce neurogenic and neuroglycopenic symptoms (50–55 mg/dL, 2.8–3.0 mmol/L) or to impair brain function in nondiabetic individuals[10,12] and substantially higher than the glucose levels that do so in people with well-controlled diabetes,[6,12] although people with poorly controlled diabetes sometimes have symptoms at somewhat higher glucose levels.[6,7]

Use of a <70 mg/dL (3.9 mmol/L) plasma glucose alert level generally gives the patient time to take action to prevent a clinical hypoglycemic episode. Also, in practice, self–plasma glucose monitoring usually is done with devices that are not precise analytical instruments, particularly at low glucose levels.[13] The recommended alert level provides some margin for their inaccuracy.

Given the therapeutic objective to reduce the frequency and the magnitude of iatrogenic hypoglycemia, people with diabetes should treat a glucose level <70 mg/dL (3.9 mmol/L).[9] The plasma glucose alert value of <70 mg/dL (3.9 mmol/L) has been cited on the websites of the U.S. Food and Drug Administration[14] and the European Medicines Agency.[15]

The plasma glucose alert value of ≤70 mg/dL (≤3.9 mmol/L) has been criticized as being too high because glucose levels are occasionally lower than that in individuals without diabetes, and its use would lead to an overestimation of the frequency of clinically important hypoglycemia.[6] The former is true, especially in women and children. The latter criticism is wide of the mark. The issue is not to estimate the frequency of clinically important hypoglycemia. It is to prevent clinically important hypoglycemia. Notably, after criticizing the ADA recommended alert value, Amiel and colleagues[6] recommended a lower limit of the therapeutic plasma glucose concentration of 72–81 mg/dL (4.0–4.5 mmol/L). Thus, there is really rather little disagreement on this ostensibly contentious issue.[16]

Classification of Hypoglycemia

The ADA Workgroup[1] and the ADA/Endocrine Society Workgroup[2] also recommended a classification of hypoglycemia in diabetes (Table 5.1). That

Table 5.1—American Diabetes Association Workgroup on Hypoglycemia Classification of Hypoglycemia in People with Diabetes

Severe hypoglycemia. An event requiring assistance of another person to actively administer carbohydrate, glucagon, or other resuscitative actions. Plasma glucose measurements may not be available during such an event, but neurological recovery attributable to the restoration of plasma glucose to normal is considered sufficient evidence that the event was induced by a low plasma glucose concentration.
Documented symptomatic hypoglycemia. An event during which typical symptoms of hypoglycemia are accompanied by a measured plasma glucose concentration ≤70 mg/dL (≤3.9 mmol/L).
Asymptomatic hypoglycemia. An event not accompanied by typical symptoms of hypoglycemia but with a measured plasma glucose concentration ≤70 mg/dL (≤3.9 mmol/L).
Probable symptomatic hypoglycemia. An event during which symptoms typical of hypoglycemia are not accompanied by a plasma glucose determination but that was presumably caused by a plasma glucose concentration ≤70 mg/dL (≤3.9 mmol/L).
Relative (or pseudo-) hypoglycemia. An event during which the person with diabetes reports any of the typical symptoms of hypoglycemia and interprets those as indicative of hypoglycemia, with a measured plasma glucose concentration >70 mg/dL (>3.9 mmol/L) but approaching that level.

Source: American Diabetes Association Workgroup on Hypoglycemia.[1]

includes severe hypoglycemia (using a definition that has been used widely since the initial report of the Diabetes Control and Complications Trial),[17] documented symptomatic hypoglycemia, and asymptomatic hypoglycemia, as well as probable symptomatic hypoglycemia and relative hypoglycemia. The latter category, also termed pseudohypoglycemia,[2] reflects the fact that patients with poorly controlled diabetes can experience symptoms of hypoglycemia as their plasma glucose concentrations fall into the physiological range.[6,7] The definition of severe hypoglycemia becomes problematic in young children with diabetes because they often need assistance with management of any hypoglycemia.

Quantitation of Hypoglycemia Unawareness

Hypoglycemia unawareness, or impaired awareness of hypoglycemia (IAH) to account for the spectrum from normal awareness through reduced awareness to complete unawareness,[18] is a component of hypoglycemia-associated autonomic failure (HAAF; see Chapter 3) and a risk factor for iatrogenic hypoglycemia (see Chapter 4). Three methods have been used to attempt to systematically identify affected patients. The method of Gold et al.[19] asks the patient to complete a seven-point scale ranging from 1, always aware, to 7, never aware, in response to the question, "Do you know when your hypos are commencing?" A score of ≥4 is considered to indicate impaired awareness of hypoglycemia. The method of Clarke et al.[20] asks eight questions about the patient's hypoglycemia experience. A score of ≥4 is considered to indicate impaired awareness of hypoglycemia. A score of ≤2 is considered to indicate awareness of hypoglycemia, leaving a score of 3 as not classifiable. The method of Pedersen-Bjergaard et al.[21] asks the patient to select one of the terms "always," "usually," "occasionally," or "never" in response to the question, "Do you recognize symptoms, when you have a hypo?" Subjects who answer "always" are classified as having normal awareness, those answering "usually" as having impaired awareness, and those answering "occasionally" or "never" as being unaware. Thus, the method of Gold et al.[19] classifies patients as being aware or having impaired awareness, that of Clarke et al.[20] also classifies patients as being aware or having impaired awareness but leaves some patients not classified, and the method of Pedersen-Bjergaard et al.[21] classifies patients as being aware, having impaired awareness, or being unaware (see Table 5.2).

An analysis of the application of all three methods to 372 patients within T1D[22] is shown in Table 5.2. Patients with impaired awareness or unawareness

Table 5.2—Proportion of 372 patients with Type 1 Diabetes Classified as Having Intact Awareness of Hypoglycemia (Aware), Impaired Awareness of Hypoglycemia (Impaired Awareness), or Hypoglycemia Unawareness (Unaware), Using Three Methods

Method	Aware	Impaired awareness	Unaware
A. Gold et al.[19]	75%	25%	–
B. Clarke et al.[20]	51%	28% (21% not classified)	–
C. Pedersen-Bjergaard[21]	41%	46%	13%

Source: Høi-Hansen et al.[22]

by all three methods reported *1*) fewer neurogenic, but not neuroglycopenic, symptoms of hypoglycemia; *2*) symptoms at lower self-monitored plasma glucose concentrations; and *3*) higher rates of severe iatrogenic hypoglycemia. Compared with those with awareness, patients classified as having impaired awareness of hypoglycemia by the methods of Gold et al.,[19] Clarke et al.,[20] and Pedersen-Bjergaard et al.[21] reported threefold, sixfold, and eightfold higher rates of severe hypoglycemia, respectively. Those classified as unaware by the method of Pederson-Bjergaard et al.[21] reported a 21-fold higher rate of severe hypoglycemia. Thus, all three methods identify patients at increased risk of severe iatrogenic hypoglycemia. The methods of Gold et al.[19] and of Petersen-Bjergaard[21] offer simplicity. Because impaired awareness or unawareness is an inducible and reversible phenomenon (see Chapter 3), none of the rather diverse proportions shown in Table 5.2 should be taken too literally, and the syndrome cannot be assumed to be stable.

Quantitation of Endogenous Insulin Deficiency

Normally, insulin secretion adapts to maintain plasma glucose concentrations within, or return them to, the postabsorptive physiological range. Insulin is secreted from pancreatic β-cells into the hepatic portal venous circulation, and ~50% is cleared by the liver. C-peptide, the peptide cleaved from proinsulin to yield insulin, is secreted in equimolar quantities with insulin. But C-peptide is not cleared by the liver. Therefore, plasma C-peptide concentrations provide an index of endogenous insulin secretion. Indeed, plasma C-peptide data can be used to calculate rates of insulin secretion.[23–25]

Plasma C-peptide concentrations are ~0.5–1.5 ng/mL (~0.2–0.5 nmol/L) after an overnight fast in healthy euglycemic individuals. Normally, the concentrations decrease as plasma glucose levels decline within the physiological range and become virtually indistinguishable from zero if glucose levels fall below the physiological range.[25]

One approach to the quantitation of endogenous insulin deficiency is to define the plasma C-peptide concentrations that identify patients with clinical T1D. In general, fasting plasma C-peptide concentrations ≤0.6 ng/mL (≤0.2 nmol/L) characterize T1D,[26–29] although a higher cutoff value has been reported[30] (see Table 5.3). A wider range of glucagon-stimulated plasma C-peptide levels has been reported to identify T1D (Table 5.3).[26–28,30]

Table 5.3—Fasting, Stimulated*, Random Plasma C-Peptide Concentrations in Patients Judged Clinically to Have Type 1 Diabetes

DCCT[26]	≤0.6 ng/mL	≤1.5 ng/mL	—
	≤0.2 nmol/L	≤0.5 nmol/L	—
Gjessing et al.[27]	<0.6 ng/mL	<1.0 ng/mL	—
	<0.2 nmol/L	<0.3 nmol/L	—
Service et al.[28]	<0.5 ng/mL	↑ <0.2 ng/mL	—
	<0.2 nmol/L	↑ <0.1 nmol/L	—
Jones & Hattersley[29]	<0.75 ng/mL	—	—
	<0.25 nmol/L	—	—
Berger et al.[30]	≤1.2 ng/mL	≤1.8 ng/mL	≤1.5 ng/mL
	≤ 0.4 nmol/L	≤0.6 nmol/L	≤0.5 nmol/L

*Stimulated patients were tested 6 min after 1.0 mg of glucagon intravenously.

Interestingly, among the 262 patients judged clinically to have type 2 diabetes (T2D) by Service et al.,[28] 20 (8%) displayed an insulin-deficient plasma C-peptide pattern initially, and an additional 33 (13%) did so on at least one occasion during subsequent testing. Unfortunately, the proportion of those patients who had late-onset autoimmune diabetes (i.e., T1D), as opposed to progression of T2D to absolute endogenous insulin deficiency, is not known.

Absolute insulin deficiency and the resulting absence of a decrease in insulin secretion (and of an increase in glucagon secretion) is a fundamental feature of defective glucose counterregulation and thus HAAF (see Chapter 3) and is a risk factor for iatrogenic hypoglycemia (see Chapter 4). A subset of patients with T1D retain some, albeit still subnormal, insulin secretion. That is relevant to defense against falling plasma glucose concentrations. For example, the proportion of patients who suffered severe hypoglycemia in the DCCT was about 50% lower in the 11% of the patients who had plasma C-peptide concentrations >0.6 ng/mL (0.2 nmol/L) during a mixed meal at baseline and at least 1 year later.[31]

References

1. American Diabetes Association Workgroup on Hypoglycemia. Defining and reporting hypoglycemia in diabetes. *Diabetes Care* 2005;28:1245–1249

2. Seaquist ER, Anderson J, Childs B, Cryer P, Dagogo-Jack S, Fish L, Heller SR, Rodriguez H, Rosenzweig J, Vigersky R. Hypoglycemia and diabetes: a report of a workgroup of the American Diabetes Association and the Endocrine Society. *Diabetes Care* 2013;36:1384–1395

3. Heller SR, Cryer PE. Reduced neuroendocrine and symptomatic responses to subsequent hypoglycemia after one episode of hypoglycemia in nondiabetic humans. *Diabetes* 1991;40:223–226

4. Fanelli CG, Dence CS, Markham J, Videen TO, Paramore DS, Cryer PE, Powers WJ. Blood-to-brain glucose transport and cerebral glucose metabolism are not reduced in poorly controlled type 1 diabetes. *Diabetes* 1998;47: 1444–1450

5. Davis SN, Shavers C, Mosqueda-Garcia R, Costa F. Effects of differing antecedent hypoglycemia on subsequent counterregulation in normal humans. *Diabetes* 1997;46:1328–1335

6. Amiel SA, Sherwin RS, Simonson DC, Tamborlane WV. Effect of intensive insulin therapy on glycemic thresholds for counterregulatory hormone release. *Diabetes* 1988;37:901–907

7. Boyle PJ, Schwartz NS, Shah SD, Clutter WE, Cryer PE. Plasma glucose concentrations at the onset of hypoglycemic symptoms in patients with poorly controlled diabetes and in nondiabetics. *N Engl J Med* 1988;318:1487–1492

8. Mitrakou A, Fanelli C, Veneman T, Perriello G, Calderone S, Platanisiotis D, Rambotti A, Raptis S, Brunetti P, Cryer P, Gerich J, Bolli G. Reversibility of unawareness of hypoglycemia in patients with insulinoma. *N Engl J Med* 1993; 329:834–839

9. International Hypoglycaemia Study Group. Minimizing hypoglycemia in diabetes. *Diabetes Care* 2015;38:1583–1591

10. Cryer PE. The prevention and correction of hypoglycemia. In *Handbook of Physiology.* Section 7, The Endocrine System. Vol. II, The Endocrine Pancreas and Regulation of Metabolism. Jefferson LS, Cherrington AD, Eds. New York, Oxford University Press, 2001, p. 1057–1092

11. Cox DJ, Gonder-Frederick LA, Kovatchev BP, Julian DM, Clarke WL. Progressive hypoglycemia's impact on driving simulation performance. *Diabetes Care* 2000;23:163–170

12. Cryer PE. Hypoglycemia, functional brain failure, and brain death. *J Clin Invest* 2007;117:868–870

13. Diabetes Research in Children Network (DirecNet) Study Group. A multicenter study of the accuracy of the One Touch Ultra home glucose meter in children with type 1 diabetes. *Diabetes Technol Ther* 2003;5:933–941

14. U.S. Department of Health and Human Services Food and Drug Administration Center for Drug Evaluation and Research (CDER). Diabetes mellitus: developing drugs and therapeutic biologics for treatment and prevention (I:\7630dft.doc). 13 February 2008. Retrieved from http://www.fda.gov/downloads/Drugs/Guidances/ucm071624.pdf

15. Committee for Medicinal Products for Human Use (CHMP). Guideline on clinical investigation of medicinal products in the treatment or prevention of diabetes mellitus CPMP/EWP/1080/00 Rev. 1, 2012. Available from http://www.ema.europa.eu/docs/en_GB/document_library/Scientific_guideline/2012/06/WC500129256.pdf. Accessed 8 February 2016

16. Cryer PE. Preventing hypoglycaemia: what is the appropriate glucose alert value? *Diabetologia* 2009;52:35–37

17. Diabetes Control and Complications Trial Research Group (DCCT). The effect of intensive treatment of diabetes on the development and progression of long-term complications in insulin dependent diabetes mellitus. *N Engl J Med* 1993;329:977–986

18. Frier BM, Fisher BM. Impaired hypoglycemia awareness. In *Hypoglycaemia in Clinical Diabetes.* Fisher BM, Frier BM, Eds. Chichester, U.K., John Wiley & Sons, 1999, p. 111–146

19. Gold AE, MacLeod KM, Frier BM. Frequency of severe hypoglycemia in patients with type 1 diabetes and impaired awareness of hypoglycemia. *Diabetes Care* 1994;17:697–703

20. Clarke WL, Cox DJ, Gonder-Frederick LA, Julian D, Schlundt D, Polonsky W. Reduced awareness of hypoglycemia in IDDM adults: a prospective study of hypoglycemia frequency and associated symptoms. *Diabetes Care* 1995;18:517–522

21. Pedersen-Bjergaard U, Pramming S, Thorsteinsson B. Recall of severe hypoglycemia and self-estimated state of awareness in type 1 diabetes. *Diabetes Metab Res Rev* 2003;19:232–240

22. Høi-Hansen T, Pedersen-Bjergaard U, Andersen RD, Kristensen PL, Thomsen C, Kjær T, Høgenhaven H, Smed A, Holst JJ, Dela F, Boomsma F, Thorsteinsson B.

Cognitive performance, symptoms and counter-regulation during hypoglycaemia in patients with type 1 diabetes and high or low renin-angiotensin system activity. *J Renin Angiotensin Aldosterone Syst* 2009;10:216–229

23. Eaton RP, Allen RC, Schade DS, Erickson KM, Standefer J. Prehepatic insulin production in man: kinetic analysis using peripheral connecting peptide behavior. *J Clin Endocrinol Metab* 1980;51:520–528

24. Polonsky KS, Licinio-Paixao J, Given BD, Pugh W, Rue P, Galloway J, Karrison T, Frank B. Use of biosynthetic human C-peptide in the measurement of insulin secretion rates in normal volunteers and type I diabetic patients. *J Clin Invest* 1986;77:98–105

25. Heller SR, Cryer PE. Hypoinsulinemia is not critical to glucose recovery from hypoglycemia in humans. *Am J Physiol Endocrinol Metab* 1991;261:E41–E48

26. Diabetes Control and Complications Trial Research Group (DCCT). The Diabetes Control and Complications Trial: design and methodologic considerations for the feasibility phase. *Diabetes* 1986;35:530–545

27. Gjessing HJ, Matzen LE, Faber OK, Frølund A. Fasting plasma C-peptide, glucagon stimulated plasma C-peptide and urinary C-peptide in relation to clinical type of diabetes. *Diabetologia* 1989;32:305–311

28. Service FJ, Rizza RA, Zimmerman BR, Dyck PJ, O'Brien PC, Melton LJ III. The classification of diabetes by clinical and C-peptide criteria. *Diabetes Care* 1997;20:198–201

29. Jones AG, Hattersley AT. The clinical utility of C-peptide measurement in the care of patients with diabetes. *Diabet Med* 2013;30:803–817

30. Berger B, Stenström G, Sundkvist G. Random C-peptide in the classification of diabetes. *Scand J Clin Lab Invest* 2000;60:687–694

31. Steffes MW, Sibley S, Jackson M, Thomas W. β-cell function and the development of diabetes related complications in the Diabetes Control and Complications Trial. *Diabetes Care* 2003;26:832–836

6
The Prevention and Treatment of Hypoglycemia in Diabetes

Prevention of Hypoglycemia: Hypoglycemia Risk Factor Reduction

It is preferable to prevent, rather than to treat, hypoglycemia in people with diabetes. The prevention of hypoglycemia requires the practice of hypoglycemia risk factor reduction (Table 6.1).[1–8] The International Hypoglycaemia Study Group[9] recommended that for patients with diabetes who are at risk of hypoglycemia as a result of treatment with a sulfonylurea, a glinide, or insulin, the diabetes health-care provider should ensure the following. First, they should *1*) acknowledge the reality or the possibility of hypoglycemia and, if hypoglycemia is a problem, consider each of the risk factors for hypoglycemic (Chapter 4), including those based on therapeutic hyperinsulinemia and those indicative of hypoglycemia-associated autonomic failure (HAAF); and *2*) apply the principles of glycemic control that are relevant to minimize the risk of hypoglycemia. Second, providers should ensure that such patients *1*) are educated about hypoglycemia, *2*) treat self-monitored plasma glucose (SMPG) or continuous glucose monitoring (CGM) glucose levels ≤70 mg/dL (≤ 3.9mmol/L) to avoid progression to clinical iatrogenic hypoglycemia, and *3*) are queried regularly about their awareness of hypoglycemia, including the glucose level at which symptoms develop. Third, in addition to drug selection

DOI: 10.2337/9781580406499.06

(i.e., avoidance of a sulfonylurea, or a glinide, use of more physiological insulin replacement and of insulin analoges) and, in selected capable and motivated patients, consideration of diabetes treatment technologies (e.g., continuous subcutaneous insulin infusion [CSII], real-time CGM, and combination of CSII and CGM ranging from sensor-augmented pump therapy to closed loop insulin, or insulin plus glucagon, replacement), providers should appreciate the relevant principles of glycemic control, including *1*) selection of individualized glycemic goals,[3,10] 2) provision of structured patient education that generally reduces the frequency of hypoglycemia,[11–15] and, typically, 3) short-term scrupulous avoidance of hypoglycemia that often reverses impaired awareness of hypoglycemia (Table 6.1).[16–19]

Acknowledge the Problem

The issue of hypoglycemia should be addressed in every contact with sulfonylurea-, glinide-, or insulin-treated people with diabetes. Patient concerns about the reality or even the possibility of hypoglycemia can be a barrier to glycemic control.[20–22] Indeed, some studies suggest that people with insulin-treated diabetes are more concerned about the possibility of an episode of hypoglycemia than about the long-term complications of diabetes.[20,23] Yet, patients are often reluctant to volunteer their concerns. They should be given the explicit opportunity to do so. It also often is helpful to question close associates of the patient, as they may have observed clues to episodes of hypoglycemia not recognized by the patient. Even if no concerns are expressed, examination of the self–plasma glucose monitoring record (or CGM data) often will disclose that hypoglycemia is a problem.

Table 6.1—Hypoglycemia Risk Factor Reduction

1. Acknowledge the problem
2. Consider the risk factors
3. Apply the relevant principles of aggressive glycemic therapy
   a. Drug selection
   b. Diabetes treatment technologies
   c. Individualized glycemic goals
   d. Structured patient education
   e. Short-term scrupulous avoidance of hypoglycemia

Consider the Risk Factors

In a patient with diabetes treated with a sulfonylurea, a glinide, or insulin in whom hypoglycemia becomes a problem, each of the risk factors for hypoglycemia discussed in Chapter 4 (see Table 4.1) should be considered carefully and the therapeutic regimen should be adjusted appropriately. Sometimes there is a straightforward solution to the problem. The conventional risk factors, based on absolute or relative insulin excess, include the dose, type, and timing of insulin or insulin secretagogue medications and the conditions in which exogenous glucose delivery or endogenous glucose production is decreased, glucose utilization or sensitivity to insulin is increased, or insulin clearance is reduced. The risk factors indicative of HAAF include the degree of absolute endogenous insulin deficiency; a history of severe hypoglycemia or impaired awareness of hypoglycemia, or both; and a relationship between hypoglycemic episodes and recent antecedent hypoglycemia, sleep, or prior exercise; and lower A1C levels. Unless the cause is easily remediable, a history of severe hypoglycemia should prompt consideration of a fundamental regimen adjustment. Without that adjustment, the risk of another episode of severe hypoglycemia is high.[24–28] Indeed, increasing nonsevere hypoglycemia predicts the occurrence of severe hypoglycemia.

Apply the Principles of Aggressive Glycemic Therapy

In general, diabetes treatment regimens should be designed to minimize hypoglycemia as well as hyperglycemia.[9] From the perspective of hypoglycemia, the therapeutic objective is to minimize the number of episodes of hypoglycemia and their severity and duration without producing hyperglycemia and raising A1C levels. Indeed, the goal is to reduce both hypoglycemia and hyperglycemia as reflected in the A1C. The principles of aggressive glycemic therapy relevant to reducing hypoglycemia include drug selection, selected use of diabetes technologies, individualized glycemic goals, structured patient education, and short-term scrupulous avoidance of hypoglycemia (Table 6.1).

Drug Selection

Drug selection to minimize the risk of hypoglycemia includes the avoidance of sulfonylurea and glinides, oral agents that can cause hypoglycemia because they stimulate insulin secretion even at normal glucose concentrations.[29] Nonetheless, sulfonylureas are inexpensive and widely available.

Among the commonly used sulfonylureas, glyburide (glibenclamide) is most often associated with hypoglycemia.[30,31] In addition, higher mortality has been reported in patients with diabetes and myocardial infarction who were treated with glyburide compared with those treated with glimepiride or gliclazide.[32] Epidemiologic data suggest that all cause mortality[33,34] and cardiovascular mortality[33] are increased in sulfonylurea-treated compared with metformin-treated type 2 diabetes (T2D). The possibility of confounding, including confounding by indication, is possible. In addition, it is conceivable that metformin might have a protective effect. As noted earlier, metformin, glucagon-like peptide-1 (GLP-1) receptor agonists, dipeptidyl peptidase-IV (DPP-IV) inhibitors, sodium-glucose cotransporter 2 (SGLT2) inhibitors, thiazolidinediones, and α-glucosidase inhibitors should not, and probably do not, cause hypoglycemia.[35–37] That is true even for GLP-1 receptor agonists and DPP-IV inhibitors, which are, among other mechanisms, insulin secretagogues. Unlike sulfonylureas, they produce glucose-dependent insulin secretion that disengages as plasma glucose concentrations fall into the normal range. All six categories of these drugs that should not cause hypoglycemia when used alone or in combination among themselves would be expected, by lowering glucose levels, to increase the risk of hypoglycemia caused by a sulfonylurea, a glinide, or insulin. The bile acid sequestrant colesevelam and the dopamine receptor agonist bromocriptine[38,39] should not cause hypoglycemia. Among potential future drugs, glucokinase activators will cause hypoglycemia.[40,41] Indeed, glucokinase activators reduce glucagon secretory responses to hypoglycemia,[42] probably because they raise intraislet insulin.[43]

In addition to more physiological insulin replacement,[44] the use of insulin analogues reduces the frequency at least of nocturnal hypoglycemia,[45,46] including severe nocturnal hypoglycemia.[47] The use of a long-acting basal insulin analogue (e.g., glargine or detemir), compared with NPH insulin, in a multiple daily injection (MDI) insulin regimen reduces the incidence of nocturnal hypoglycemia, perhaps that of total and symptomatic hypoglycemia, in type 1 diabetes (T1D) and T2D.[46,48–53] Compared with insulin glargine, among the newer long-acting basal insulins,[54] insulin degludec reduced confirmed nocturnal hypoglycemia in T1D[55] and confirmed and overall hypoglycemia in T2D[56]; insulin glargine 300 units/mL reduced nocturnal hypoglycemia, including severe hypoglycemia, in T2D[57]; and insulin peglispro reduced nocturnal hypoglycemia in T1D[58] and T2D.[59] (Compared with human regular insulin, the use of a rapid-acting prandial insulin (lispro, aspart, or glulisine) reduces the incidence of nocturnal hypoglycemia at least in T1D.[45,48,49,60] A basal-bolus MDI regimen (i.e., a basal long-acting insulin coupled with a prandial rapid-acting insulin, as needed) has been reported to produce the lowest mean glycemia and rates of hypoglycemia compared with biphasic insulin twice daily or prandial insulin alone.[61] GLP-1 receptor agonists also inhibit glucagon secretion in a glucose-dependent fashion. They decrease glucagon secretion during hyperglycemia and euglycemia, but not during hypoglycemia. Indeed, they may enhance glucagon secretion during hypoglycemia.[62] Interestingly, combined basal insulin plus GLP-1 receptor agonist therapy has been reported to reduce hypoglycemia when compared with basal-bolus insulin therapy in T2D.[63]

Diabetes Technologies

Diabetes treatment technologies include CSII, CGM, and combinations of CSII and CGM, which ultimately lead to closed-loop insulin (or insulin and glucagon) replacement. It seems likely that some, perhaps all, of these technologies ultimately will be shown convincingly to be beneficial to patients with T1D and advanced T2D. That judgment will be based on compelling evidence that the technology improves glycemic control (typically assessed with A1C) without increasing hypoglycemia (or that it reduces hypoglycemia without deterioration of glycemic control) and the extent to which it does so. When assessing whether the technology is clinically meaningful, issues such as impact on quality of life and cost become relevant.

Given that one can vary the rate of basal insulin subcutaneous insulin infusion throughout the 24-h period, CSII, typically with a rapid-acting insulin analogue, may be superior to MDI therapy in a basal-bolus insulin regimen in selected capable and motivated patients with T1D.[64,65] One meta-analysis of randomized controlled trials of CSII compared with MDI disclosed only a small decrease in A1C (−0.2%) with no significant decrease in severe or nocturnal hypoglycemia.[66] Another meta-analysis concluded that CSII, compared with MDI, had not been shown to reduce the incidence of hypoglycemia in T1D or T2D.[67] In general, trials comparing CSII with MDI that used an insulin analogue in the MDI regimen have found no difference in achieved A1C or in the prevalence of hypoglycemia.[68,69] A systematic review of randomized controlled trials in pregnant women with diabetes did not show a significant difference between CSII and MDI.[70]

Real-time CGM reports subcutaneous glucose concentrations, which lag changes in plasma glucose by up to 15 min, suffers from relative inaccuracy of the sensors at low glucose levels, and requires that the device be used consistently.[71,72] CGM alone has had a rather minimal effect to reduce the frequency of iatrogenic hypoglycemia.[73–75] Nonetheless, use of real-time CGM has been found to be associated with an A1C reduction in the range of 0.4 to 0.6% in adults with T1D who generally actually used the device[76–79] without a detected increase in hypoglycemia. The trials, however, were underpowered to detect an increase in hypoglycemia.[76] In another study of patients with T1D, A1C levels were 0.3% lower and glucose excursions to <63 mg/dL (<3.5 mmol/L) were reduced during the night.[73] Interestingly, real-time CGM was found to result in increased epinephrine secretory responses to hypoglycemia (i.e., to partially reverse HAAF), presumably because of less iatrogenic hypoglycemia, although that finding was not documented in patients with T1D.[80] In one study of a CGM device in patients with T1D at high risk for severe hypoglycemia, the sensitivity and specificity of the device for detecting plasma glucose concentrations <70 mg/dL (< 3.9 mmol/L) were only 65 and 80%, respectively. The sum of false positive results (15%) and false negative results (10%) was greater than the proportion of true positive results (18%).[75]

The combination of CSII and real-time CGM—that is, sensor-augmented pump therapy, particularly that including an insulin pump programmed to suspend insulin infusion for up to 2 h when CGM glucose levels fall to a selected low glucose value—has been reported to reduce the frequency of severe hypoglycemia in T1D.[81–83] Although an earlier meta-analysis concluded that neither real-time CGM (compared with SMPG) or sensor-augmented pump therapy (compared with MDI and SMG) had been shown to reduce the incidence of hypoglycemia,[67] both CSII and CGM have been associated with a reduced frequency of severe hypoglycemia.[84] In the hypoglycemia beneficial HypoCOMPaSS trial,[14] neither CSII (compared with MDI) nor CGM (compared with SMPG) reduced severe hypoglycemia or improved awareness of hypoglycemia to a greater extent.

Fully closed-loop insulin[85] or insulin and glucagon[86] replacement and pancreatic islet transplantation,[87] like successful pancreas transplantation, undoubtedly will eliminate hypoglycemia when these become consistently successful. Despite its theoretical advantages, clear evidence that closed-loop insulin plus glucagon, compared with insulin alone, replacement remains to be established convincingly.[88] Successful islet (or pancreas) transplantation eliminates hypoglycemia as long as the graft survives sufficiently to permit independence from insulin injections.[89] Interestingly, even after a requirement for insulin therapy recurs, only partial graft function is required to suppress severe hypoglycemia,[87] whereas greater graft function is required to abrogate hyperglycemia.[90] That observation underscores the key role of a decrease in insulin levels in the prevention of hypoglycemia (see Chapter 2). Successful islet transplantation partially restores decrements in insulin and increments in glucagon, epinephrine, symptoms, and endogenous glucose production during hypoglycemia.[91] Finally, glucagon receptor antagonists have been reported to lower plasma glucose concentrations in several experimental diabetes animal models[92] and humans with T2D[93] without hypoglycemia.

Special circumstances relevant to drug selection and technologies associated with the prevention of hypoglycemia in diabetes include exercise, the overnight fast, older age, driving, and pregnancy. Especially in insulin-treated patients, hypoglycemia can occur during or shortly after exercise[94] or late after exercise.[95,96] The latter is the result of exercise-associated HAAF.[97–100] Because it often occurs at night (following afternoon exercise), hypoglycemia also can be the result of sleep-associated HAAF (see Chapter 3).[101–103] Measures to avoid early-onset exercise hypoglycemia include interspersing episodes of intense exercise (which tends to raise plasma glucose concentrations), adding carbohydrate ingestion (e.g., 1.0 $g \cdot kg^{-1} \cdot h^{-1}$), and reducing insulin doses.[104] With respect to the latter, a reduction of pre- and postexercise premeal rapid-acting insulin doses reduced early-onset but not late-onset hypoglycemia in patients with T1D.[105] Adolescents with T1D have been found to require higher rates of glucose infusion to maintain euglycemia during raised, but constant, insulin infusions and fasting for more than 11 h after midday exercise than after midday rest, perhaps reflecting restoration of muscle and hepatic glucogen stores.[106]

A consistent observation since the DCCT[24,107,108] is that more than half of episodes of hypoglycemia, including severe hypoglycemia, occur during the night.[109,110] That is typically the longest interval between meals and between SMPG and includes the time of maximal sensitivity to insulin. In addition to the use of insulin analogues,[46,48–52] sensor-augmented pump therapy, or closed-loop insulin replacement, approaches to the prevention of nocturnal hypoglycemia include attempts to produce sustained delivery of exogenous carbohydrate or sustained endogenous glucose production throughout the night.[71] With respect to the former approach, a conventional bedtime snack or bedtime administration of uncooked cornstarch have not been found to be consistently effective[71] as the duration of their glycemic action is too short. With respect to the latter approach, bedtime administration of 5 mg of the epinephrine-simulating β_2–adrenergic agonist terbutaline has been shown to prevent nocturnal hypoglycemia in adults with aggressively treated T1D, albeit at the expense of hyperglycemia the following morning.[71] A 2.5-mg bedtime dose of terbutaline produced intermediate results on nocturnal plasma glucose levels without morning hyperglycemia.[111] The higher plasma glucose concentrations following terbutaline were likely the result of β_2–adrenergic stimulations of hepatic and renal glucose production, but they also may have been the result of β_2–adrenergic stimulation at a ventromedial hypothalamic site with subsequent sympathoadrenal, at least adrenomedullary, epinephrine and α-cell glucagon secretion.[112] Inhaled formoterol, another β_2–adrenergic agonist, raises plasma glucose concentrations in patients with T2D.[113] An alternative approach to decreasing nocturnal hypoglycemia in patients using CSII is to reduce the basal insulin infusion rate at bedtime. A comparison of *1*) a 20% reduction in insulin dose at bedtime, *2*) a 2.5-mg dose of terbutaline at bedtime, and *3*) no treatment at bedtime in children with T1D disclosed that the reduction in insulin dose and terbutaline administration resulted in comparable hyperglycemia during the night, but terbutaline more consistently prevented nocturnal hypoglycemia.[114] These, and other potentially effective treatments, have been reviewed.[115,116] Parenthetically, there is now considerable evidence against the Somogyi hypothesis[117]; morning hyperglycemia is the result of the lack of insulin and not of posthypoglycemic insulin resistance.[118–120] There is a dawn phenomenon—a growth hormone–mediated increase in the nighttime to morning plasma glucose concentration[121]—but its magnitude is small.[122]

Glucose counterregulatory defenses against falling plasma glucose concentrations are impaired minimally by age per se.[123,124] Nonetheless, diabetes is increasingly common in older individuals and that includes the transition of T2D to absolute endogenous insulin deficiency and all of the resulting pathophysiology (see Chapter 3) and risk factors for hypoglycemia (see Chapter 4) discussed earlier. In addition to HAAF, comorbidities including renal insufficiency, polypharmacy, and impaired cognition all were relevant in older individuals.[125,126] Also, the issue of relative benefit from glycemic control comes into play. The incidence of hypoglycemia increases with the duration of diabetes and age. It is difficult to separate the effects of these, but it appears both are involved.[127] Drivers with diabetes and a history of recurrent hypoglycemia-related driving mishaps have been found to have more symptoms during euglycemia (i.e., more symptom "noise"), greater driving-simulator impairments, and fewer intense hormonal counterregulatory responses to hypoglycemia.[128,129] Obviously, SMPG (or attention to CGM values) is critical before performance of any critical task, including driving, particularly for individuals with impaired awareness of hypoglycemia. Additionally, up to 45% of pregnant women with T1D experience severe hypoglycemia with substantially higher rates in the first trimester.[130] Hypoglycemia also occurs in insulin-treated pregnant women with T2D.[131] Some evidence suggests that pregnancy is associated with suppression of glucose counterregulation.[132]

Individualized Glycemic Goals

There is consensus that glycemic goals should be individualized in patients with diabetes.[3,10,133] Given the evidence that glycemic control partially prevents or delays microvascular complications of diabetes and may partially prevent or delay macrovascular complications, it follows that a lower A1C is in the best interest of people with diabetes if that can be achieved and maintained safely. Thus, a reasonable individualized glycemic goal is the lowest A1C that does not cause severe hypoglycemia (that requiring the assistance of another person) and preserves awareness of hypoglycemia, preferably with little or no symptomatic or even asymptomatic hypoglycemia, at a given stage in the evolution of the individual's diabetes.[3] Thus, the glycemic goal should be linked not only to the mean level of glycemic control (i.e., the A1C) but also to the risk of hypoglycemia, specifically to the drugs used, the degree of endogenous insulin deficiency, and the hypoglycemia history, as well as the anticipated benefit of the targeted level of glycemic control. Action is required when a sulfonylurea, glinide, or insulin regimen causes severe hypoglycemia, impaired awareness of hypoglycemia, or an unacceptable number of symptomatic or asymptomatic hypoglycemic episodes.

In a patient with T2D treated effectively with lifestyle changes or drugs that do not cause hypoglycemia, a normal A1C is a reasonable generic goal. Conversely, in an older patient with diabetes and a limited life expectancy, an A1C just sufficient to prevent symptoms of hyperglycemia is reasonable. There is evidence of glycemic overtreatment of older adults with diabetes who are unlikely to benefit from tight glycemic control.[134,135]

While still recommending a glycemic goal of an A1C <7.0% (<53 mmol/mol) for most adults with diabetes, or of <7.5% (<58 mmol/mol) for those <18 years of age,[136] the American Diabetes Association and the European Association for the Study of Diabetes have recommended individualized glycemic goals for people with diabetes.[10,133] They suggest that less stringent A1C goals—7.5 to 8.0% (58 to 64 mmol/mol), or even slightly higher—are appropriate for patients with a history of severe hypoglycemia. Target A1C recommendations are based on epidemiological data.[3,61,137,138] Notably, an analysis of A1C data from patients with T1D from the Swedish National Diabetes Register indicated that adjustment for time-updated status with respect to renal disease yielded risk estimates for both death from any cause and death from cardiovascular causes that were virtually unchanged for patients with A1C levels ranging from 7.0 to 7.8% (53 to 61 mmol/mol) versus A1C levels of 6.9% (52 mmol/mol) or lower.[139] Individualized glycemic goals based on both A1C and the risk of and experience with hypoglycemia have been reviewed.[3]

Structured Patient Education

The core approach, applicable to virtually all patients with diabetes treated with a sulfonylurea, a glinide, or insulin in whom hypoglycemia becomes a problem, is achieved through structured patient education (often re-education) that teaches the patient how and when their drugs can cause hypoglycemia; how to adjust their medications, meal plans, and exercise to optimize glycemic control and minimize hypoglycemia; and how to recognize and treat hypoglycemia.[9] Based conceptually on earlier inpatient education programs,[11] there is increasing empirical evidence that such structured outpatient education decreases hypoglycemia, and often with a decrease in A1C.[12–15,140] For example, a structured education program in flexible insulin therapy led to a reduction of impaired awareness of hypoglycemia (45% of those with impaired awareness initially were aware at 1 year) and a reduction in severe hypoglycemia (from 1.9 to 0.6 episodes per patient-year) and a small but significant decrease in A1C in patients with T1D.[12] Patient education needs to cover a broad range of information and skill training and often needs to include a motivational element.[9]

In addition to basic diabetes teaching, patients with diabetes treated with a sulfonylurea, a glinide, or insulin should receive structured education about hypoglycemia and how to avoid it. They need to be taught about the anticipation, recognition, and treatment of hypoglycemia. They need to know the common symptoms of hypoglycemia; and, over time, they need to understand their individual most meaningful symptoms, how to document hypoglycemia with SMPG, and how to treat (and not overtreat) hypoglycemia. Close associates need to be taught how to recognize severe hypoglycemia and how to prepare and administer glucagon. Patients need to understand the risk factors for hypoglycemia (Table 4.1), including the effects of the dose and timing of their individual secretagogue or insulin preparations, as well as the effects of missed meals and the overnight fast, alcohol, and exercise. With respect to the latter, patients used strategies to defend against planned or unanticipated exercise. They also need to know that episodes of hypoglycemia signal an increased likelihood of future, often more severe, episodes.

Short-Term Scrupulous Avoidance of Hypoglycemia

In patients with impaired awareness of hypoglycemia, structured patient education should be combined with 2 to 3 weeks of scrupulous avoidance of hypoglycemia—which may require acceptance of somewhat higher glycemic goals in the short term—because that higher goal can be expected to restore awareness in most affected patients.[16–19] People with diabetes treated with a sulfonylurea, a glinide, or insulin should be educated about hypoglycemia, should treat SMPG (or CGM) glucose levels to <70 mg/dL (<3.9 mmol/L) to avoid progression to clinical iatrogenic hypoglycemia, and should be queried regularly about hypoglycemia, including the SMPG (or CGM) level at which symptoms develop.[9]

Treatment of Hypoglycemia

Hypoglycemia causes functional brain failure that is corrected in the vast majority of instances after the plasma glucose concentration is raised.[141] Profound and prolonged hypoglycemia can cause brain death but most fatal episodes are the result of other mechanisms, presumably ventricular arrhythmias (see Chapter 3). Clearly, the plasma glucose concentration should be raised to normal levels promptly. Data from rodent models of extreme hypoglycemia suggest that post-treatment hyperglycemia may contribute to neuronal death.[141,142] In one study in rats, there was more neuronal necrosis in the hippocampus and greater mortality when the posthypoglycemic blood glucose concentration was raised to >162 mg/dL (9.0 mmol/L) but not when the posthypoglycemic value was less than that.[143] Indeed, evidence shows that posthypoglycemia hyperglycemia increases measures of endothelial damage and thrombosis activation in individuals without diabetes and in those with T1D.[144] Thus, it appears that posthypoglycemia hyperglycemia should be avoided.

In people with diabetes, most episodes of asymptomatic hypoglycemia (detected by SMPG or CGM) or of mild-to-moderate symptomatic hypoglycemia are effectively self-treated by ingestion of glucose tablets or carbohydrate-containing juice, soft drinks, candy, other snacks, or a meal.[2,145,146] A reasonable dose is 20 gm of glucose (see Figure 6.1).[2,146] Clinical improvement should occur in 15–20 min. In the setting of ongoing hyperinsulinemia, however, the glycemic response to oral glucose is transient—typically <2 h.[146] Thus, ingestion of a more substantial snack or meal shortly after the plasma glucose level is raised is generally advisable. In contrast to swallowed glucose, glucose applied to the buccal mucosa is not absorbed.[147] Administration of the somatostatin analog octreotide, which inhibits insulin secretion, can be used as a supplement to glucose administration in the treatment of sulfonylurea-induced hypoglycemia.[148,149]

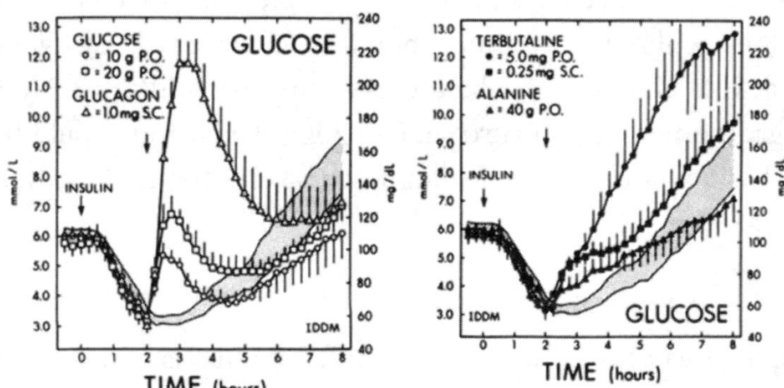

Figure 6.1— Mean (±SE) plasma glucose concentrations during insulin-induced hypoglycemia in patients with type 1 diabetes (IDD, insulin-dependent diabetes) in the absence of an intervention (shaded area) and after the indicated interventions. S.C., subcutaneous, P.O., per os.

Source: Reproduced from Wiethop and Cryer[150] with permission from the American Diabetes Association.

Parenteral treatment is required when a hypoglycemic patient is unwilling (because of neuroglycopenia) or unable to take carbohydrate orally. Glucagon, injected subcutaneously or intramuscularly in a usual dose of 1.0 mg in adults by an associate of the patient, often is used.[151] That can be lifesaving, but it often causes substantial, albeit transient, hyperglycemia (see Figure 6.1), and it can cause nausea or even vomiting. Smaller doses of glucagon (e.g., 150 µg), repeated if necessary, have been found to be effective without side effects in children.[152] The increase in endogenous glucose production in response to such microgram doses of glucagon is attenuated by increased insulin levels in patients with T1D.[153] A single dose of glucagon is sometimes ineffective, but additional glucagon administration is often effective.[154] Advances that can be anticipated include development of a glucagon that is stable in solution,[155] which would obviate the need to reconstitute the drug before its administration and would be key to the use of glucagon with insulin in a bihormonal artificial pancreas, and development of a method to deliver glucagon intranasally,[156] which would obviate the need for parenteral injection. Intranasal delivery of glucagon with a device that does not require drug reconstitution has been reported to produce increments in plasma glucose concentrations comparable to those produced by injected glucagon, but without nausea or vomiting.[156] Because it stimulates insulin secretion, glucagon might be less useful in patients other than those with T1D or advanced T2D. Indeed, glucagon has been reported to cause hypoglycemia in individuals without diabetes.[157,158] Because it acts primarily by stimulating hepatic glycogenolysis, glucagon treatment is ineffective in glycogen-depleted individuals (e.g., after a binge of alcohol ingestion).

Although glucagon can be administered intravenously by medical personnel, in that setting, intravenous glucose is the standard parenteral therapy. A common initial dose of intravenous glucose is 25 g,[2,145] but lower doses could be used in a setting in which plasma glucose concentrations can be measured serially. The glycemic response to intravenous glucose is transient in the setting of ongoing hyperinsulinemia. A subsequent glucose infusion often is needed, and food should be provided as soon as the patient is able to ingest it safely.

The duration of a hypoglycemic episode is a function of its cause. An episode caused by a rapid-acting insulin secretagogue or insulin analog will be relatively brief, whereas that caused by a long-acting insulin analog will be substantially longer. A sulfonylurea overdose, or that of a long-acting insulin analog, can result in prolonged hypoglycemia requiring hospitalization.

Clinical Practice Guidelines

Many of the principles discussed in this book were incorporated, by a panel organized by the Endocrine Society, into a set of clinical practice guidelines for the evaluation and management of adult hypoglycemic disorders.[158] The development of the guidelines included an assessment of the strength of the supporting evidence, resulting in suggestions based on

Table 6.2—Clinical Practice Guidelines

1. We suggest that individuals with diabetes become concerned about the possibility of developing hypoglycemia when the self-monitored blood glucose concentration is falling rapidly or is <70 mg/dl (<3.9 mmol/l).
2. Given the established long-term microvascular, and potential macrovascular, benefits of glycemic control, we recommend that the therapeutic glycemic goal be the lowest mean glycemia (e.g., A1C) that can be accomplished safely in a given patient at a given point in the progression of that individual patient's diabetes.
3. We recommend that the prevention of hypoglycemia in diabetes involves addressing the issue in each patient contact and, if hypoglycemia is a problem, making adjustments in the regimen based on review and application of the principles of aggressive glycemic therapy—patient education and empowerment, frequent self blood glucose monitoring, flexible and appropriate insulin or insulin secretagogue regimens, individualized glycemic goals, and ongoing professional guidance and support—and consideration of each of the known risk factors for hypoglycemia.
4. We recommend that both the conventional risk factors and those indicative of compromised defenses against hypoglycemia be considered in a patient with recurrent treatment-induced hypoglycemia. The conventional risk factors are excessive or ill-timed dosing of, or wrong type of, insulin or insulin secretagogue and conditions under which exogenous glucose delivery or endogenous glucose production is decreased, glucose utilization is increased, sensitivity to insulin is increased, or insulin clearance is decreased. Compromised defenses against hypoglycemia are indicated by the degree of endogenous insulin deficiency, a history of severe hypoglycemia or hypoglycemia unawareness or both, as well as recent antecedent hypoglycemia, prior exercise or sleep, and lower glycemic goals per se.
5. With a history of hypoglycemia unawareness (i.e., recurrent hypoglycemia without symptoms), we recommend a 2- to 3-week period of scrupulous avoidance of hypoglycemia, with the anticipation that awareness of hypoglycemia will return in many patients.
6. Unless the cause is easily remediable, we recommend that an episode of severe hypoglycemia should lead to a fundamental review of the treatment regimen.
7. We recommend that urgent treatment of hypoglycemia should be accomplished by ingestion of carbohydrates if that is feasible and by parenteral glucagon or glucose if the former is not feasible.

Source: Cryer et al.[158]

weaker evidence and recommendations based on stronger evidence. The suggestions and recommendations concerning hypoglycemia in people with diabetes are listed in Table 6.2. The American Diabetes Association and the Endocrine Society have also addressed the issue of hypoglycemia in diabetes.[159]

References

1. Cryer PE, Davis SN, Shamoon H. Hypoglycemia in diabetes. *Diabetes Care* 2003;26:1902–1912
2. Cryer PE. The barrier of hypoglycemia in diabetes. *Diabetes* 2008;57: 3169–3176
3. Cryer PE. Glycemic goals in diabetes: trade-off between glycemic control and iatrogenic hypoglycemia. *Diabetes* 2014;63:2188–2195
4. Cryer PE. Hypoglycemia. In *Williams Textbook of Endocrinology*. 13th ed. Melmed S, Polonsky KS, Larsen PR, Kronenberg HM, Eds. Philadelphia, Elsevier, 2016, p. 1582–1607
5. Rossetti P, Porcellati F. Prevention of hypoglycemia while achieving good glycemic good glycemic control in type 1 diabetes. Diabetes Care 2008;31(Suppl. 2): S113–S120
6. Amiel SA, Dixon T, Mann R, Jameson K. Hypoglycaemia in type 2 diabetes. *Diabet Med* 2008;25:245–254
7. Amiel SA. Hypoglycemia: from the laboratory to the clinic. *Diabetes Care* 2009;32:1364–1371
8. Graveling AJ, Frier BM. Hypoglycaemia: an overview. *Primary Care Diabetes* 2009;3:131–139
9. International Hypoglycaemia Study Group. Minimizing hypoglycemia in diabetes. *Diabetes Care* 2015;38:1583–1591
10. Inzucchi SE, Bergenstal RM, Buse JB, Diamant M, Ferrannini E, Nauck M, Peters AL, Tsapas A, Wender R, Matthews DR. Management of hyperglycemia in type 2 diabetes, 2015: a patient centered approach; update to a position statement of the American Diabetes Association (ADA) and the European Association for the Study of Diabetes (EASD). *Diabetes Care* 2015;38:140–149
11. Sämann A, Mühlhauser I, Bender R, Kloos CH, Müller UA. Glycaemic control and severe hypoglycaemia following training in flexible, intensive insulin therapy

to enable dietary freedom in people with type 1 diabetes: a prospective implementation study. *Diabetologia* 2005;48:1965–1970

12. Hopkins D, Lawrence I, Mansell P, Thompson G, Amiel S, Campbell M, Heller S. Improved biomedical and psychological outcomes 1 year after structured education in flexible insulin therapy for people with type 1 diabetes: the U.K. DAFNE experience. *Diabetes Care* 2012;35:1638–1642

13. de Zoysa N, Rogers H, Stadler M, Gianfrancesco C, Beveridge S, Britneff E, Choudhary P, Elliott J, Heller S, Amiel SA. A psychoeducational program to restore hypoglycemia awareness: the DAFNE-HART pilot study. *Diabetes Care* 2014;37:863–866

14. Little SA, Leelarathna L, Walkinshaw E, Tan HK, Chapple O, Lubina-Solomon A, Chadwick TJ, Barendse S, Stocken DD, Brennand C, Marshall SM, Wood R, Speight J, Kerr D, Flanagan D, Heller SR, Evans ML, Shaw JAM. Recovery of hypoglycemia awareness in long-standing type 1 diabetes: a multicenter 2 X 2 factorial randomized controlled trial comparing insulin pump with multiple daily injections and continuous with conventional glucose self-monitoring (HypoCOMPaSS). *Diabetes Care* 2014;37:2114–2122

15. Elliott J, Jacques RM, Kruger J, Campbell MJ, Amiel SA, Mansell P, Speight J, Brennan A, Heller SR. Substantial reductions in the number of diabetic ketoacidosis and severe hypoglycaemia episodes requiring emergency treatment lead to reduced costs after structured education in adults with type 1 diabetes. *Diabet Med* 2014;31:847–853

16. Fanelli CG, Epifano L, Rambotti AM, Pampanelli S, Di Vincenzo A, Modarelli F, Lepore M, Annibale B, Ciofetta M, Bottini P, Porcellati F, Scionti L, Santeusanio F, Brunetti P, Bolli GB. Meticulous prevention of hypoglycemia normalizes the glycemic thresholds and magnitude of most of neuroendocrine responses to, symptoms of, and cognitive function during hypoglycemia in intensively treated patients with short-term IDDM. *Diabetes* 1993;42:1683–1689

17. Fanelli C, Pampanelli S, Epifano L, Rambotti AM, Di Vincenzo A, Modarelli F, Ciofetta M, Lepore M, Annibale B, Torlone E, Perriello G, De Feo P, Santeusanio F, Brunetti P, Bolli GB. Long-term recovery from unawareness, deficient counterregulation and lack of cognitive dysfunction during hypoglycemia, following institution of rational, intensive therapy in IDDM. *Diabetologia* 1994;37:1265–1276

18. Cranston I, Lomas J, Maran A, Macdonald I, Amiel SA. Restoration of hypoglycaemia awareness in patients with long-duration insulin-dependent diabetes. *Lancet* 1994;344:283–287

19. Dagogo-Jack S, Rattarasarn C, Cryer PE. Reversal of hypoglycemia unawareness, but not defective glucose counterregulation, in IDDM. *Diabetes* 1994;43: 1426–1434

20. Nordfeldt S, Ludvigsson J. Fear and other disturbances of severe hypoglycaemia in children and adolescents with type 1 diabetes mellitus. *J Pediatr Endocrinol Metab* 2005;18:83–91

21. Wild D, von Maltzahn R, Brohan E, Christensen T, Clausen P, Gonder-Frederick L. A critical review of the literature on fear of hypoglycemia in diabetes: implications for diabetes management and patient education. *Patient Educ Couns* 2007;68:10–15

22. Gonder-Frederick L. Fear of hypoglycemia: a review. *Diabetic Hypoglycemia* 2013;5:3–11

23. Pramming S, Thorsteinsson B, Bendtson I, Binder C. Symptomatic hypoglycaemia in 411 type 1 diabetic patients. *Diabet Med* 1991;8:217–222

24. Diabetes Control and Complications Trial Research Group (DCCT). Hypoglycemia in the Diabetes Control and Complications Trial. *Diabetes* 1997;46:271–286

25. Kovatchev BP, Cox DJ, Gonder-Frederick LA, Young-Hyman D, Schlundt D, Clarke WL. Assessment of risk for severe hypoglycemia among adults with IDDM: validation of the low blood glucose index. *Diabetes Care* 1998;21: 1870–1875

26. Kovatchev BP, Cox DJ, Kumar A, Gonder-Frederick LA, Clarke WL. Algorithmic evaluation of metabolic control and risk of severe hypoglycemia in type 1 and type 2 diabetes using self-monitoring blood glucose (SMBG) data. *Diabetes Technol Ther* 2003;5:817–828

27. Cox DJ, Gonder-Frederick L, Ritterband L, Clarke W, Kovatchev BP. Prediction of severe hypoglycemia. *Diabetes Care* 2007;30:1370–1373

28. Sreenan S, Andersen M, Thorsted BL, Wolden ML, Evans M. Increased risk of severe hypoglycemic events with increasing frequency of non-severe hypoglycemic events on patients with type 1 and type 2 diabetes. *Diabetes Ther* 2014;5:447–458

29. Riefflin A, Ayyagari U, Manley SE, Holman RR, Levy JC. The effect of glibenclamide on insulin secretion at normal glucose concentrations. *Diabetologia* 2015;58:43–49

30. Holstein A, Egberts EH. Risk of hypoglycaemia with oral antidiabetic agents in patients with type 2 diabetes. *Exp Clin Endocrinol Metab* 2003;111:405–414

31. Gangji AS, Cukierman T, Gerstein HC, Goldsmith GH, Clase CM. A systematic review and meta-analysis of hypoglycemia and cardiovascular events. *Diabetes Care* 2007;30:389–394

32. Zeller M, Danchin N, Simon D, Vahanian A, Lorgis L, Cottin Y, Berland J, Gueret P, Wyart P, Deturck R, Tabone X, Machecourt J, Leclercq F, Drouet E, Mulak G, Bataille V, Cambou JP, Ferrieres J, Simon T, and the French Registry of Acute ST-Elevation and Non-ST-Elevation Myocardial Infarction investigators. Impact of type of preadmission sulfonylureas on mortality and cardiovascular outcomes in diabetic patients with acute myocardial infarction. *J Clin Endocrinol Metab* 2008;95:4993–5002

33. Evans JM, Ogston SA, Emslie-Smith A, Morris AD. Risk of mortality and adverse cardiovascular outcomes in type 2 diabetes: a comparison of patients treated with sulfonylureas and metformin. *Diabetologia* 2006;49:930–936

34. Tzoulaki I, Molokhia M, Curcin V, Little MP, Millett CJ, Ng A, Hughes RI, Khunti K, Wilkins MR, Majeed A, Elliott P. Risk of cardiovascular disease and all cause mortality among patients with type 2 diabetes prescribed oral antidiabetes drugs: retrospective cohort study using UK general practice research database. *BMJ* 2009;339:b4731

35. Ferrannini E, Ramos SJ, Salsali A, Tang W, List JF. Dapagliflozin monotherapy in type 2 diabetic patients with inadequate glycemic control by diet and exercise. A randomized, double-blind, placebo-controlled, phase 3 trial. *Diabetes Care* 2010;33:2217–2224

36. Tschope D, Bramlage P, Binz C, Krekler M, Plate T, Deeg E, Gitt AK. Antidiabetic pharmacotherapy and anamnestic hypoglycemia in a large cohort of type 2 diabetic patients an analysis of the DiaRegis registry. *Cardiovasc Diabetol* 2011;10:66

37. Mearns ES, Sobieraj DM, White CM, Saulsberry WJ, Kohn CG, Doleh Y, Zaccaro E, Coleman CI. Comparative efficacy and safety of antidiabetic drug regimens added to metformin monotherapy in patients with type 2 diabetes: a network meta-analysis. *PLoS One* 2015;10:e0125879

38. Gaziano JM, Cincotta AH, O'Connor CM, Ezrokhi M, Rutty D, Ma ZJ, Scranton RE. Randomized clinical trial of quick-release bromocriptine among patients with type 2 diabetes on overall safety and cardiovascular outcomes. *Diabetes Care* 2010;33:1503–1508

39. DeFronzo RA. Bromocriptine: a sympatholytic, D2-dopamine agonist for the treatment of type 2 diabetes [published correction appears in *Diabetes Care* 2011;34:1442]. *Diabetes Care* 2011;34:789–794

40. Matschinsky FM, Zelent B, Doliba N, Li C, Vanderkooi JM, Naji A, Sarabu R, Grimsby J. Glucokinase activators for diabetes therapy. *Diabetes Care* 2011; 34(Suppl. 2):S236–S243

41. Meininger GE, Scott R, Alba M, Shentu Y, Luo E, Amin H, Davies MJ, Kaufman KD, Goldstein BJ. Effects of MK-0941, a novel glucokinase activator, on glycemic control in insulin-treated patients with type 2 diabetes. *Diabetes Care* 2011;34:2560–2566

42. Norjavaara E, Ericsson H, Sjoberg F, Leonsson-Zachrisson M, Sjostrand M, Morrow LA, Hompesch M. Glucokinase activators AZD6370 and AZD1656 do not affect the central counterregulatory response to hypoglycemia in healthy males. *J Clin Endocrinol Metab* 2012;97:3319–3325

43. Cooperberg BA, Cryer PE. Insulin reciprocally regulates glucagon secretion in humans. *Diabetes* 2010;59:2936–2940

44. Amiel SA. Risks of intensive therapy. In *Hypoglycemia in Clinical Diabetes*, 3rd ed. Chichester, U.K., Wiley-Blackwell, 2014, p. 145–164

45. Siebenhofer A, Plank J, Berghold A, Jeitler K, Horvath K, Narath M, Gfrerer R, Pieber TR. Short acting insulin analogues versus regular human insulin in patients with diabetes mellitus. *Cochrane Database Syst Rev* 2006;2:CD003287. http://www.ncbi.nlm.nih.gov/pubmed/16625575

46. Horvath K, Jeitler K, Berghold A, Ebrahim SH, Gratzer TW, Plank J, Kaiser T, Pieber TR, Siebenhofer A. Long-acting insulin analogues versus NPH insulin (human isophane insulin) for type 2 diabetes. *Cochrane Database Syst Rev* 2007;2:CD005613. doi:10.1002/14651858.CD005613.pub3

47. Pedersen-Bjergaard U, Kristensen PL, Beck-Nielsen H, Nørgaard K, Perrild H, Christiansen JS, Jensen T, Hougaard P, Parving HH, Thorsteinsson B, Tarnow L. Effect of insulin analogues on risk of severe hypoglycemia (HypoAna Trial): a prospective, randomized, open-label, blinded-endpoint crossover trial. *Lancet Diabetes Endocrinol* 2014;2:553–561

48. Hirsch IB. Insulin analogues. *N Engl J Med* 2005;352:174–183

49. Gough SCL. A review of human and analogue insulin trials. *Diabetes Res Clin Pract* 2007;77:1–15

50. Monami M, Marchionni N, Mannucci S. Long-acting insulin analogues vs. NPH human insulin in type 1 diabetes: a meta-analysis. *Diabetes Obes Metab* 2009; 11:372-378

51. Little S, Shaw J, Home P. Hypoglycemia rates with basal insulin analogs. *Diabetes Technol Ther* 2011;13(Suppl. 1):S53–S64

52. Rosenstock J, Fonseca V, Schinzel S, Dain MP, Mullins P, Riddle M. Reduced risk of hypoglycemia with once-daily glargine versus twice-daily NPH and number needed to harm with NPH to demonstrate the risk of one additional hypoglycemic event in type 2 diabetes: evidence from a long-term controlled trial. *J Diabetes Complications* 2014;28:742–749

53. Tricco AC, Ashoor HM, Antony J, Beyene J, Veroniki AA, Isaranuwatchai W, Harrington A, Wilson C, Tsouros S, Soobiah C, Yu CH, Hutton B, Hoch JS, Hemmelgarn BR, Moher D, Majumdar SR, Strauss SE. Safety, effectiveness and cost effectiveness of long acting versus intermediate acting insulin for patients with type 1 diabetes: systematic review and network meta-analysis. *BMJ* 2014;349:g5459

54. Bolli GB, DeVries JH, New long-acting insulin analogs: from clamp studies to clinical practice. *Diabetes Care* 2015;38:541–543.

55. Heller S, Buse J, Fisher M, Garg S, Marre M, Merker L, Renard E, Russell-Jones D, Philotheou A, Francisco AMO, Pei H, Bode B, on behalf of the BEGIN Basal-Bolus Type 1 Trial Investigators. Insulin degludec, an ultra-long-acting basal insulin, versus insulin glargine in basal-bolus treatment with mealtime insulin aspart in type 1 diabetes (Begin Basal-Bolus Type 1): a phase 3, randomised, open-label, treat-to-target non-inferiority trial. *Lancet* 2012;379:1489–1497

56. Garber AJ, King AB, Del Prato S, Sreenan S, Balci MK, Muñoz-Torres M, Rosenstock J, Endahl LA, Francisco AMO, Hollander P, on behalf of the NN1250-3582 (BEGIN BB T2D) Trial Investigators. Insulin degludec, an ultra-longacting basal insulin, versus insulin glargine in basal-bolus treatment with mealtime insulin aspart in type 2 diabetes (BEGIN Basal-Bolus Type 2): a phase 3, randomised, open-label, treat-to-target non-inferiority trial. *Lancet* 2012;379:1498–1507

57. Riddle MC, Bolli GB, Ziemen M, Muehlen-Bartmer I, Bizet F, Home PD on behalf of the EDITION 1 Study Investigators. New insulin glargine 300 units/mL versus glargine 100 units/mL in people with type 2 diabetes using basal and mealtime insulin: glucose control and hypoglycemia in a 6-month randomized controlled trial (EDITION 1). *Diabetes Care* 2014;37:2755–2762

58. Rosenstock J, Bergenstal RM, Blevins TC, Morrow LA, Prince MJ, Qu Y, Sinha VP, Howey DC, Jacober SJ. Better glycemic control and weight loss with the novel long-acting basal insulin LY2605541 compared with insulin glargine in type 1 diabetes: a randomized, crossover study. *Diabetes Care* 2013;36:522–528

59. Bergenstal RM, Rosenstock J, Arakaki RF, Prince MJ, Qu Y, Sinha VP, Howey DC, Jacober SJ. A randomized, controlled study of once-daily LY2605541, a

novel long-acting basal insulin, versus insulin glargine in basal insulin-treated patients with type 2 diabetes. *Diabetes Care* 2012;35:2140–2147

60. Heller S, Bode B, Kozlovski P, Svendsen AL. Meta-analysis of insulin aspart versus regular human insulin used in a basal-bolus regimen for the treatment of diabetes mellitus. *J Diabetes* 2013;5:482–491

61. Holman RR, Farmer AJ, Davies MJ, Levy JC, Darbyshire JL, Keenan JF, Paul SK, for the 4-T Study Group. Three-year efficacy of complex insulin regimens in type 2 diabetes. *N Engl J Med* 2009;361:1736–1747

62. Dunning BS, Foley JS, Ahrén B. Alpha cell function in health and disease: influence of glucagon-like peptide-1. *Diabetologia* 2005;48:1700–1713

63. Eng C, Kramer CK, Zinman B, Retnakaran R. Glucagon-like peptide-1 receptor agonist and basal insulin combination treatment for the management of type 2 diabetes: a systematic review and meta-analysis. *Lancet* 2014;384:2228–2234

64. Cooper MN, O'Connell SM, Davis EA, Jones TW. A population-based study of risk factors for severe hypoglycaemia in a contemporary cohort of childhood-onset type 1 diabetes. *Diabetologia* 2013;56:2164–2170

65. Johnson SR, Cooper MN, Jones TW, Davis SA. Long-term outcome of insulin pump therapy in children with type 1 diabetes assessed in a large population-based case-control study. *Diabetologia* 2013;56:2392–2400

66. Fatourechi MM, Kudva YC, Murad MH, Elamin MB, Tabini CC, Montori VM. Hypoglycemia with intensive insulin therapy. A systematic review and meta-analysis of randomized trials of continuous subcutaneous insulin infusion versus multiple daily injections. *J Clin Endocrinol Metab* 2009;94:729–740

67. Yeh HC, Brown TT, Maruthur N, Ranasinghe P, Berger Z, Suh YD, Wilson LM, Haberl EB, Brick J, Bass EB, Golden SH. Comparative effectiveness and safety of methods of insulin delivery and glucose monitoring for diabetes mellitus: a systematic review and meta-analysis. *Ann Intern Med* 2012;157: 336–347

68. Bolli GB, Kerr D, Thomas R, Torlone E, Sola-Gazagnes A, Vitacolonna E, Selam JL, Home PD. Comparison of a multiple daily insulin injection regime (basal once-daily glargine plus mealtime lispro) and continuous subcutaneous insulin infusion (lispro) in type 1 diabetes. A randomized open parallel multicenter study. *Diabetes Care* 2009;32:1170–1176

69. Cummins E, Royle P, Snaith A, Greene A, Robertson L, McIntyre L, Waugh N. Clinical effectiveness and cost-effectiveness of continuous subcutaneous insulin

infusion for diabetes: systematic review and economic evaluation. *Health Technol Assess* 2010;14:1–181

70. Mukhopadhyay A, Farrell T, Fraser RB, Ola B. Continuous subcutaneous insulin infusion vs intensive conventional insulin therapy in pregnant diabetic women: a systematic review and metaanalysis of randomized, controlled trials. *Am J Obstet Gynecol* 2007;197:447–456
71. Raju B, Arbelaez AM, Breckenridge S, Cryer PE. Noctournal hypoglycemia in type 1 diabetes: an assessment of preventative bedtime treatments. *J Clin Endocrinol Metab* 2006;91:2087–2092
72. Hermanides J, Phillip M, DeVries JH. Current application of continuous glucose monitoring in the treatment of diabetes. Pros and cons. *Diabetes Care* 2011; 34(Suppl. 2):S197–S201
73. Battelino T, Phillip M, Bratina N, Nimri R, Oskarsson P, Bolinder J. Effect of continuous glucose monitoring on hypoglycemia in type 1 diabetes. *Diabetes Care* 2011;34:795–800
74. Langendam M, Luijf YM, Hooft L, Devries JH, Mudde AH, Scholten RJ. Continuous glucose monitoring systems for type 1 diabetes mellitus. *Cochrane Database of Systemic Reviews* 2012;1:CD008101
75. Bay C, Kristensen PL, Pedersen-Bjergaard U, Tarnow L, Thorsteinsson B. Nocturnal continuous glucose monitoring: accuracy and reliability of hypoglycemia detection in patients with type 1 diabetes at high risk of severe hypoglycemia. *Diabetes Technol Ther* 2013;15:371–377
76. Juvenile Diabetes Research Foundation (JDRF) Continuous Glucose Monitoring Study Group. Continuous glucose monitoring and intensive treatment of type 1 diabetes. *N Engl J Med* 2008;359:1464–1476
77. Juvenile Diabetes Research Foundation (JDRF) Continuous Glucose Monitoring Study Group. Factors predictive of use and of benefit from continuous glucose monitoring in type 1 diabetes. *Diabetes Care* 2009;32:1947–1953
78. Juvenile Diabetes Research Foundation (JDRF) Continuous Glucose Monitoring Study Group. Sustained benefit of continuous glucose monitoring on A1C, glucose profiles, and hypoglycemia in adults with type 1 diabetes. *Diabetes Care* 2009;32:2047–2049
79. Juvenile Diabetes Research Foundation (JDRF) Continuous Glucose Monitoring Study Group. Prolonged nocturnal hypoglycemia is common during 12 months of continuous glucose monitoring in children and adults with type 1 diabetes. *Diabetes Care* 2010;33:1004–1008

80. Ly TT, Hewitt J, Davey RJ, Lim E-M, Davis EA, Jones TW. Improving epinephrine responses in hypoglycemia unawareness with real-time continuous glucose monitoring in adolescents with type 1 diabetes. *Diabetes Care* 2011;34: 50–52

81. Bergenstal RM, Klonoff DC, Garg SK, Bode BW, Meredith M, Slover RH, Ahmann AJ, Welsh JB, Lee SW, Kaufman FR, for the ASPIRE In-Home Study Group. Threshold-based insulin-pump interruption for reduction of hypoglycemia. *N Engl J Med* 2013;369:224–232

82. Ly TT, Nicholas JA, Retterath A, Lim EM, Davis EA, Jones TW. Effect of sensor-augmented insulin pump therapy and automated insulin suspension vs standard insulin pump therapy on hypoglycemia in patients with type 1 diabetes: a randomized clinical trial. *JAMA* 2013;310:1240–1247

83. Maahs DM, Calhoun P, Buckingham BA, Chase HP, Hramiak I, Lum J, Cameron F, Bequette BW, Aye T, Paul T, Slover R, Wadwa RP, Wilson DM, Kollman C, Beck RW; In Home Closed Loop Study Group. A randomized trial of a home system to reduce nocturnal hypoglycemia in type 1 diabetes. *Diabetes Care* 2014;37:1885–1891

84. Choudhary P, Ramasamy S, Green L, Gallen G, Pender S, Brackenridge A, Amiel SA, Pickup JC. Real-time continuous glucose monitoring significantly reduces severe hypoglycemia in hypoglycemia-unaware patients with type 1 diabetes. *Diabetes Care* 2013;36:4160–4162

85. Leelarathna L, Dellweg S, Mader JK, Allen JM, Benesch C, Doll W, Ellmerer M, Hartnell S, Heinemann L, Kojzar H, Michalewski L, Nodale M, Thabit H, Wilinska ME, Pieber TR, Arnolds S, Evans ML, Hovorka R, on behalf of the AP@home Consortium. Day and night home closed-loop insulin delivery in adults with type 1 diabetes: three-center randomized crossover study. *Diabetes Care* 2014;37:1931–1937

86. Russell SJ, El-Khatib FH, Sinha M, Magyar KL, McKeon K, Goergen LG, Balliro C, Hillard MA, Nathan DM, Damiano ER. Outpatient glycemic control with a bionic pancreas in type 1 diabetes. *N Engl J Med* 2014;371:313–325

87. Ang M, Meyer C, Brendel MD, Bretzel RG, Linn T. Magnitude and mechanisms of glucose counterregulation following islet transplantation in patients with type 1 diabetes suffering from severe hypoglycaemic episodes. *Diabetologia* 2014; 57:623–632

88. Haidar A, Legault L, Messier V, Mitre TM, Leroux C, Rabasa-Lhoret R. Comparison of dual-hormone artificial pancreas, single-hormone artificial pancreas,

and conventional insulin pump therapy for glycaemic control in patients with type 1 diabetes: an open-label randomised controlled crossover trial. *Lancet Diabetes Endocrinol* 2015;3:17–26

89. Ryan EA, Shandro T, Green K, Paty BW, Senior PA, Bigam D, Shapiro AM, Vantyghem MC. Assessment of the severity of hypoglycemia and glycemic lability in type 1 diabetic subjects undergoing islet transplantation. *Diabetes* 2004;53:955–962

90. Vantyghem MC, Raverdy V, Balavoine AS, Defrance F, Caiazzo R, Arnalsteen L, Gmyr V, Hazzan M, Noel C, Kerr-Conte J, Pattou F. Continuous glucose monitoring after islet transplantation in type 1 diabetes: an excellent graft function (beta-score greater than 7) is required to abrogate hyperglycemia, whereas a minimal function is necessary to suppress severe hypoglycemia (beta-score greater than 3). *J Clin Endocrinol Metab* 2012;97:E2078–2083

91. Rickels MR, Fuller C, Dalton-Bakes C, Markmann E, Palanjian M, Cullison K, Yiao J, Kapoor S, Liu C, Naji A, Teff KL. Restoration of glucose counterregulation by islet transplantation in long-standing type 1 diabetes. *Diabetes* 2015;64: 1713–1718

92. Okamoto H, Kim J, Aglione JP, Lee J, Cavino K, Na E, Rafique A, Kim JH, Harp J, Valenzuela DM, Yancopoulos GH, Murphy AJ, Gromada J. Glucagon receptor blockade with a human antibody normalizes blood glucose in diabetic mice and monkeys. *Endocrinology* 2015;156:2781–2794

93. Kelly RP, Garhyan P, Raddad E, Fu H, Lim CN, Prince MJ, Pinaire JA, Loh MT, Deeg MA. Short-term administration of glucagon receptor antagonist LY2409021 lowers blood glucose in healthy people and in those with type 2 diabetes. *Diabetes Obes Metab* 2015;17:414–422

94. Tansey MJ, Tsalikian E, Beck RW, Mauras N, Buckingham BA, Weinzimer SA, Janz KF, Kollman C, Xing D, Ruedy KJ, Steffes MW, Borland TM, Singh RJ, Tamborlane WV, for the Diabetes Research in Children Network (DirecNet) Study Group. The effects of aerobic exercise on glucose and counterregulatory hormone concentrations in children with type 1 diabetes. *Diabetes Care* 2006;29:20–25

95. MacDonald MJ. Post exercise late onset hypoglycemia in insulin-dependent diabetic patients. *Diabetes Care* 1987;10:584–588

96. Tsalikian E, Mauras N, Beck RW, Tamborlane WV, Janz KF, Chase HP, Wysocki T, Weinzimer SA, Buckingham BA, Kollman C, Xing D, Ruedy KJ, for the Diabetes Research in Network (DirecNet) Study Group. Impact of exercise on overnight glycemic control in children with type 1 diabetes. *J Pediatr* 2005;147:528–534

97. Galassetti P, Mann S, Tate D, Neill RA, Costa F, Wasserman DH, Davis SN. Effects of antecedent prolonged exercise on subsequent counterregulatory responses to hypoglycemia. *Am J Physiol Endocrinol Metab* 2001;280:E908–E917

98. Sandoval DA, Aftab Guy DL, Richardson MA, Ertl AC, Davis SN. Effects of low and moderate antecedent exercise on counterregulatory responses to subsequent hypoglycemia in type 1 diabetes. *Diabetes* 2004;53:1798–1806

99. Ertl AC, Davis SN. Evidence for a vicious cycle of exercise and hypoglycemia in type 1 diabetes mellitus. *Diabetes Metab Res Rev* 2004;20:124–130

100. Younk LM, Davis SN. Hypoglycemia and hypoglycemia unawareness during and following exercise in type 1 diabetes. In *Type 1 Diabetes: Clinical Management of the Athlete*. Gallen I, Ed. London, Springer-Verlag, 2012, p. 115–150

101. Jones TW, Porter P, Sherwin RS, Davis EA, O'Leary P, Frazer F, Byrne G, Stick S, Tamborlane WV. Decreased epinephrine responses to hypoglycemia during sleep. *N Engl J Med* 1998;338:1657–1662

102. Banarer S, Cryer PE. Sleep-related hypoglycemia-associated autonomic failure in type 1 diabetes. Reduced awakening from sleep during hypoglycemia. *Diabetes* 2003;52:1195–1203

103. Schultes B, Jauch-Chara K, Gais S, Hallschmid M, Reiprich E, Kern W, Oltmanns KM, Peters A, Fehm HL, Born J. Defective awakening response to nocturnal hypoglycemia in patients with type 1 diabetes mellitus. *PLoS Medicine* 2007; 4:e69

104. Gallen IW. Hypoglycemia associated with exercise in people with type 1 diabetes. *Diabetic Hypoglycemia* 2014;7:3–10

105. Campbell MD, Walker M, Trenell MI, Jakovljevic DG, Stevenson EJ, Bracken RM, Bain SC, West DJ. Large pre- and postexercise rapid-acting insulin reductions preserve glycemia and prevent early- but not late-onset hypoglycemia in patients with type 1 diabetes. *Diabetes Care* 2013;36:2217–2224

106. Davey RJ, Howe W, Paramalingam N, Ferreira LD, Davis EA, Fournier PA, Jones TW. The effect of midday moderate-intensity exercise on postexercise hypoglycemia risk in individuals with type 1 diabetes. *J Clin Endocrinol Metab* 2013;98:2908–2914

107. Diabetes Control and Complications Trial Research Group (DCCT). Epidemiology of severe hypoglycemia in the Diabetes Control and Complications Trial. *Am J Med* 1991;90:450–459

108. Diabetes Control and Complications Trial Research Group (DCCT). The effect of intensive treatment of diabetes on the development and progression of long-term complications in insulin dependent diabetes mellitus. *N Engl J Med* 1993;329:977–986

109. Chico A, Vidal-Rios P, Subirà M, Novials A. The continuous glucose monitoring system is useful for detecting unrecognized hypoglycemias in patients with type 1 and type 2 diabetes but is not better than frequent capillary glucose measurements for improving metabolic control. *Diabetes Care* 2003;26:1153–1157

110. Guillod L, Comte-Perret, Monbaron D, Gaillard RC, Ruiz J. Nocturnal hypoglycemia in type 1 diabetic patients: what can we learn with continuous glucose monitoring? *Diabetes Metab* 2007;33:360–365

111. Cooperberg BA, Breckenridge SM, Arbeláez AM, Cryer PE. Terbutaline and the prevention of nocturnal hypoglycemia in type 1 diabetes. *Diabetes Care* 2008;31: 2271–2272

112. Szepietowska B, Zhu W, Chan O, Horblitt A, Dziura J, Sherwin RS. Modulation of β-adrenergic receptors in the ventromedial hypothalamus influences counterregulatory responses to hypoglycemia. *Diabetes* 2011;60:3154–3158

113. Belfort-DeAguiar RD, Naik S, Hwang J, Szepietowska B, Sherwin RS. Inhaled formoterol diminishes insulin-induced hypoglycemia in type 1 diabetes. *Diabetes Care* 2015;38:1736–1741

114. Taplin CE, Cobry E, Messer L, McFann K, Chase HP, Fiallo-Scharer R. Preventing post-exercise nocturnal hypoglycemia in children with type 1 diabetes. *J Pediatr* 2010;157:784–788

115. Cryer PE. Death during intensive glycemic therapy of diabetes: mechanisms and implications. *Am J Med* 2011;124:993–996

116. Cryer PE. Mechanisms of hypoglycemia-associated autonomic failure in diabetes. *N Engl J Med* 2013;369:362–372

117. Choudhary P, Davies C, Emery CJ, Heller SR. Do high fasting glucose levels suggest nocturnal hypoglycaemia? The Somogyi effect—more fiction than fact? *Diabet Med* 2013;30:914–917

118. Havlin CE, Cryer PE. Nocturnal hypoglycemia does not result commonly in major morning hyperglycemia in patients with diabetes mellitus. *Diabetes Care* 1987;10:141–147

119. Tordjman KM, Havlin CE, Levandoski LA, White NH, Santiago JV, Cryer PE. Failure of nocturnal hypoglycemia to cause fasting hyperglycemia in patients with insulin-dependent diabetes mellitus. *N Engl J Med* 1987;317:1552–1559

120. Hirsch IB, Smith LJ, Havlin CE, Shah SD, Clutter WE, Cryer PE. Failure of nocturnal hypoglycemia to cause daytime hyperglycemia in patients with IDDM. *Diabetes Care* 1990;13:133–142

121. Campbell PJ, Bolli GB, Cryer PE, Gerich JE. Pathogenesis of the dawn phenomenon in patients with insulin-dependent diabetes mellitus. *N Engl J Med* 1985;312:1473–1479

122. Perriello G, De Feo P, Torlone E, Fanelli C, Santeusanio F, Brunetti P, Bolli GB. The dawn phenomenon in type 1 (insulin-dependent) diabetes mellitus: magnitude, frequency, variability, and dependency on glucose counterregulation and insulin sensitivity. *Diabetologia* 1991;34:21–28

123. Marker JC, Cryer PE, Clutter WE. Attenuated glucose recovery from hypoglycemia in the elderly. *Diabetes* 1992;41:671–678

124. Meneilly GS, Cheung E, Tuokko H. Altered responses to hypoglycemia of healthy elderly people. *J Clin Endocrinol Metab* 1994;78:1341–1348

125. Alagiakrishnan K, Mereu L. Approach to managing hypoglycemia in elderly patients with diabetes. *Postgrad Med* 2010;122:129–137

126. Kirkman MS, Briscoe VJ, Clark N, Florez H, Haas LB, Halter JB, Huang ES, Korytkowski MT, Munshi MN, Odegard PS, Pratley RE, Swift CS. Diabetes in older adults. *Diabetes Care* 2012;35:2650–2664

127. Huang ES, Laiteerapong N, Liu JY, John PM, Moffet HH, Karter AJ. Rates of complications and mortality in older diabetes patients:the diabetes and aging study. *JAMA Intern Med* 2014;174:251–258

128. Cox DJ, Kovatchev BP, Anderson SM, Clarke WL, Gonder-Frederick LA. Type 1 diabetic drivers with and without a history of recurrent hypoglycemia-related driving mishaps. Physiological and performance differences during euglycemia and the induction of hypoglycemia. *Diabetes Care* 2010;33:2430–2435

129. Cox DJ, Singh H, and Lorber D. Diabetes and driving safety: science, ethics, legality and practice. *Am J Med Sci* 2013;345:263–265

130. Nielsen LR, Pedersen-Bjergaard U, Thorsteinsson B, Johansen M, Damm P, Mathiesen ER. Hypoglycemia in pregnant women with type 1 diabetes. *Diabetes Care* 2008;31:9–14

131. Secher AL, Mathiesen ER, Andersen HU, Peter D, Lene R. Severe hypoglycemia in pregnant women with type 2 diabetes—a relevant clinical problem. *Diabetes Res Clin Pract* 2013;102:e17–18

132. Rosenn BM, Miodovnik M, Khoury JC, Siddiqi TA. Counterregulatory hormonal responses to hypoglycemia during pregnancy. *Obstet Gynecol* 1996;87: 568–574

133. Inzucchi SE, Bergenstal RM, Buse JB, Diamant M, Ferrannini E, Nauck M, Peters AL, Tsapas A, Wender R, Matthews DR. Management of hyperglycemia in type 2 diabetes: a patient-centered approach: position statement of the American Diabetes Association (ADA) and the European Association for the Study of Diabetes (EASD). *Diabetes Care* 2012; 35:1364–1379

134. Tseng C-L, Soroka O, Maney M, Aron DC, Pogach LM. Assessing potential glycemic overtreatment in persons at hypoglycemic risk. *JAMA Intern Med* 2014; 174:259–268

135. Lipska KJ, Ross JS, Miao Y, Shah ND, Lee SJ, Steinman MA. Potential overtreatment of diabetes mellitus in older adults with tight glycemic control. *JAMA Intern Med* 2015. doi:10.1001/jamainternmed.2014.7345

136. Chiang JL, Kirkman MS, Laffel LMB, Peters AL, on behalf of the Type 1 Diabetes Sourcebook Authors. Type 1 diabetes through the life span: a position statement of the American Diabetes Association. *Diabetes Care* 2014;37: 2034–2054

137. Diabetes Control and Complications Trial/Epidemiology of Diabetes Interventions and Complications (DCCT/EDIC) Research Group. Intensive diabetes treatment and cardiovascular disease in patients with type 1 diabetes. *N Engl J Med* 2005;353:2643–2653

138. Diabetes Control and Complications Trial/Epidemiology of Diabetes Interventions and Complications (DCCT/EDIC) Research Group. Association between 7 years of intensive treatment of type 1 diabetes and long-term mortality. *JAMA* 2015;313:45–53

139. Lind M, Svensson AM, Kosiborod M, Gudbjørnsdottir S, Pivodic A, Wedel H, Dalquist S, Clements M, Rosengren A. Glycemic control and excess mortality in type 1 diabetes. *N Engl J Med* 2014;371:1972–1982

140. Leelarathna L, Little SA, Walkinshaw E, Tan HK, Lubina-Solomon A, Kumareswaran K, Lane AP, Chadwick T, Marshall SM, Speight J, Flanagan D, Heller SR,

Shaw JA, Evans ML. Restoration of self-awareness of hypoglycemia in adults with long-standing type 1 diabetes: hyperinsulinemic-hypoglycemic clamp substudy results from the HypoCOMPaSS trial. *Diabetes Care* 2013;36: 4063–4070

141. Cryer PE. Hypoglycemia, functional brain failure, and brain death. *J Clin Invest* 2007;117:868–870

142. Suh SW, Gum ET, Hamby AM, Chan PH, Swanson RA. Hypoglycemic neuronal death is triggered by glucose reperfusion and activation of neuronal NADPH oxidase. *J Clin Invest* 2007;117:910–918

143. Chu X, Zhao Y, Liu F, Mi Y, Shen J, Wang X, Liu J, Jin W. Rapidly raised blood sugar will aggravate brain damage after severe hypoglycemia in rats. *Cell Biochem Biophys* 2014;69:131–139

144. Ceriello A, Novials A, Ortega E, La Sala L, Pujadas G, Testa R, Bonfigli AR, Esposito K, Giugliano D. Evidence that hyperglycemia after recovery from hypoglycemia worsens endothelial function and increases oxidative stress and inflammation in healthy control subjects and subjects with type 1 diabetes. *Diabetes* 2012;61:2993–2997

145. MacCuish AC. Treatment of hypoglycemia. In *Diabetes and Hypoglycemia.* Frier BM, Fisher BM, Eds. London, Edward Arnold, 1993, p. 212–221

146. Wiethop BV, Cryer PE. Glycemic actions of alanine and terbutaline in IDDM. *Diabetes Care* 1993;16:1124–1130

147. Gunning RR, Garber AJ. Bioactivity of instant glucose. Failure of absorption through oral mucosa. *JAMA* 1978;240:1611–1612

148. Boyle PJ, Justice K, Krentz AJ, Nagy RJ, Schade DS. Octreotide reverses hyperinsulinemia and prevents hypoglycemia induced by sulfonylurea overdoses. *J Clin Endocrinol Metab* 1993;76:752–756

149. Dougherty PP, Lee SC, Lung D, Klein-Schwartz W. Evaluation of the use and safety of octreotide as antidotal therapy for sulfonylurea overdose in children. *Pediatr Emerg Care* 2013;29:292–295

150. Wiethop BV, Cryer PE. Alanine and terbutaline in the treatment of hypoglycemia in IDDM. *Diabetes Care* 1993;16:1131–1136

151. Kedia N. Treatment of severe diabetic hypoglycemia with glucagon: an underutilized therapeutic approach. *Diabetes Metab Syndr Obes* 2011;4:337–346

152. Haymond MW, Schreiner B. Mini-dose glucagon rescue to children with type 1 diabetes. *Diabetes Care* 2001;24:643–645

153. Youssef JE, Castle JR, Bakhtiani PA, Haidar A, Branigan DL, Breen M, Ward WK. Quantification of the glycemic response to microdoses of subcutaneous glucagon at varying insulin levels. *Diabetes Care* 2014;37:3054–3060

154. Boido A, Ceriani V, Pontiroli AE. Glucagon for hypoglycemia episodes in insulin treated diabetic patients: a systematic review and meta-analysis with a comparison of glucagon with dextrose and different glucagon formulations. *Acta Diabetol* 2015;52:405–412

155. Chabenne J, Chabenne MD, Zhao Y, Levy J, Smiley D, Gelfanov V, Dimarchi R. A glucagon analog chemically stabilized for immediate treatment of life-threatening hypoglycemia. *Mol Metab* 2014;3:293–300

156. Pontiroli AE. Intranasal glucagon: a promising approach for treatment of severe hypoglycemia. *J Diabetes Sci Technol* 2015;9:38–43

157. Murad MH, Coto-Yglesias F, Wang AT, Sheidaee N, Mullan RJ, Elamin MB, Erwin PJ, Montori VM. Drug-induced hypoglycemia: a systemic review. *J Clin Endocrinol Metab* 2009;94:741–745

158. Cryer PE, Axelrod L, Grossman AB, Heller SR, Montori VM, Seaquist ER, Service FJ. Evaluation and management of adult hypoglycemic disorders. *J Clin Endocrinol Metab* 2009;94:709–728

159. Seaquist ER, Anderson J, Childs B, Cryer PE, Dagogo-Jack S, Fish L, Heller SR, Rodriguez H, Rosenzweig J, Vigersky R. Hypoglycemia and diabetes: a report of a workgroup of the American Diabetes Association and the Endocrine Society. *Diabetes Care* 2013;36:1384–1395

7
Perspective on Hypoglycemia in Diabetes

Diabetes is an increasingly common chronic disease. Its human and economic costs are large and, despite advances in therapy, these costs are growing because of the increasing prevalence of diabetes. Since the introduction of insulin therapy in 1922, it has been possible to prevent early death from diabetic ketoacidosis or hyperosmolar coma and to eliminate symptoms of uncontrolled hyperglycemia in the vast majority of patients. By the mid-20th century it was apparent that the early insulin therapies did not prevent the long-term microvascular and macrovascular complications of diabetes. Diabetes became the leading cause of end-stage renal disease requiring dialysis or transplantation, of blindness with its onset in working-age adults, and of nontraumatic amputations, and most people with diabetes died from cardiovascular disease. There were important practical advances in diabetes care in the late 20th century. Those included the development of A1C measurements to quantitate overall glycemic control, self–plasma glucose monitoring (and, more recently, continuous glucose monitoring) to assess short-term glycemic control, insulin analogs with more favorable (albeit less than ideal) pharmacokinetic profiles, an array of new drugs that lower plasma glucose concentrations early in the course of type 2 diabetes (T2D), and the concept of a diabetes care team, among other advances. Since the landmark Diabetes Control and Complications Trial in type 1 diabetes (T1D), published in 1993,[1] many studies, including the U.K. Prospective Diabetes Study in T2D,[2]

DOI: 10.2337/9781580406499.07

have led to widespread consensus that long-term glycemic control partially prevents or delays at least the microvascular complications of diabetes. Nonetheless, microvascular and macrovascular complications are still a reality for many people with diabetes. Furthermore, the impact of the barrier of iatrogenic hypoglycemia, the limiting factor in the glycemic management of many people with diabetes, has been more widely appreciated (see Chapter 1).

Glycemic control, which is the focus of this book because its topic is hypoglycemia in diabetes, is but one aspect of the management of diabetes. For example, it is now clear that blood lipid and blood pressure control, as well as blood glucose control, are fundamentally important to the prevention or delay of the vascular complications of diabetes. Although it is now possible to drive low-density lipoprotein (LDL) cholesterol to subphysiological levels and to normalize blood pressure pharmacologically, usually without major side effects, in the vast majority of people with diabetes, it is still not possible to maintain euglycemia over a lifetime of diabetes because of the barrier of iatrogenic hypoglycemia. Weight reduction and smoking cessation are often additional relevant challenges.

On the basis of insight into the physiology of glucose counterregulation (see Chapter 2) and its pathophysiology in diabetes, as well as the relationship of the latter to clinical hypoglycemia (see Chapter 3), many risk factors for iatrogenic hypoglycemia have been identified (see Chapter 4) and a working definition and classification of hypoglycemia in diabetes has been proposed (see Chapter 5). Thus, it is now possible to both improve glycemic control and reduce the risk of hypoglycemia in many people with diabetes (see Chapter 6). As developed in Chapter 6, the risk of hypoglycemia is not nonmodifiable.[3–5]

It is important for both diabetes health-care providers and people with diabetes to keep the problem of iatrogenic hypoglycemia in perspective. The underlying principle of the glycemic management of diabetes is that maintenance of glycemia as close to the nondiabetic range as can be accomplished safely over time is in the patient's best interests. It reduces the development of microvascular complications and may reduce macrovascular complications as well. The extent to which that goal can be met is a function of many factors, including the type of diabetes and the stage in the evolution of diabetes in an individual patient. T2D is, by far, the more common type of diabetes. Early in the course of T2D, hyperglycemia may respond to lifestyle changes, specifically weight loss, or to plasma glucose–lowering drugs that do not raise circulating insulin levels and therefore should not, and probably do not, cause hypoglycemia. Those include the biguanide metformin, thiazolidinediones, α-glucosidase inhibitors, and sodium-glucose cotransporter 2 (SGLT2) inhibitors that do not cause hyperinsulinemia. They also include glucagon-like peptide-1 (GLP-1) receptor agonists and dipeptidyl peptidase-IV (DPP-IV) inhibitors, which raise insulin levels only in the presence of hyperglycemia. In theory, when such drugs are effective, there is no reason not to accelerate their dosing until euglycemia is achieved in the absence of nonglycemic side effects. The reality, however, is that either initially, or over time, as patients with T2D become progressively more endogenous insulin deficient, these drugs (even in combination) fail to provide glycemic control. Insulin secretagogues, a sulfonylurea or a glinide, are also effective early in the course of T2D, although these raise endogenous insulin levels and therefore introduce the possibility of iatrogenic hypoglycemia. Ideally, they should be avoided, but the sulfonylureas remain inexpensive. Nonetheless, as emphasized in Chapter 1, the frequency of iatrogenic hypoglycemia is relatively low (at least with current glycemic goals) during treatment with an insulin secretagogue, or even with insulin, early in the course of T2D when glucose counterregulatory defenses are intact. Thus, over most of the course of the most common type of diabetes, it is possible to achieve a meaningful degree of glycemic control without risk or with relatively low risk of iatrogenic hypoglycemia. Clearly, that is beneficial to those patients. Therefore, it is fundamentally important that concerns about the risk of hypoglycemia should not be used as an excuse for poor glycemic control by diabetes health-care providers or by people with diabetes in most instances. Rather, both should strive to achieve and maintain the greatest glycemic control that can be accomplished safely in a given patient with diabetes at a given stage of his or her diabetes.

All people with T1D, and ultimately many people with T2D, require treatment with insulin. Insulin is demonstrably effective. Given in sufficient doses, it will lower plasma glucose concentrations in virtually all people with diabetes. Insulin therapy is life-saving in T1D and is necessary in those with advanced (i.e., absolutely insulin deficient) T2D. In the latter patients, it should be introduced earlier, rather than later, when other therapies fail to achieve glycemic control. The difficulty is that, although it is demonstrably effective, insulin is not demonstrably safe. Because of the pharmacokinetic and pharmacodynamic imperfections of insulin therapy, particularly in the setting of compromised glucose counterregulation (the syndromes of defective glucose counterregulation and hypoglycemia unawareness and therefore hypoglycemia-associated autonomic failure) that develops early in T1D and later in T2D, it is limited by the barrier of iatrogenic hypoglycemia. Therefore, the goal of long-term euglycemia is not feasible in such patients with current insulin regimens.

Although it can be minimized in many patients, the problem of iatrogenic hypoglycemia in T1D and advanced T2D has not been solved. Diabetes will someday be cured and prevented, but no one knows when that will be accomplished. Short of a cure, elimination of hypoglycemia from the lives of people with diabetes likely will be accomplished by the development of methods that provide plasma glucose–regulated insulin replacement (i.e., closed-loop insulin therapy or insulin plus glucagon) or secretion (i.e., implantation of insulin-secreting cells or expansion of β-cell mass). In the meantime, innovative research, ranging from studies of the fundamental molecular and cellular mechanisms of the physiology and pathophysiology of glucose counterregulation to clinical trials of novel approaches to the prevention of iatrogenic hypoglycemia, clearly is needed if we are to improve the lives of all people affected by diabetes by eliminating hypoglycemia.

References

1. Diabetes Control and Complications Trial Research Group (DCCT). The effect of intensive treatment of diabetes on the development and progression of long-term complications in insulin dependent diabetes mellitus. *N Engl J Med* 1993;329:977–986

2. United Kingdom Prospective Diabetes Study 24: A 6-year, randomized, controlled trial comparing sulfonylurea, insulin, and metformin therapy in patients with newly diagnosed type 2 diabetes that could not be controlled with diet therapy. *Ann Intern Med* 1998;128:165–175

3. Inzucchi SE, Bergenstal RM, Buse JB, Diamant M, Ferrannini E, Nauck M, Peters AL, Tsapas A, Wender R, Matthews DR. Management of hyperglycemia in type 2 diabetes: a patient-centered approach: position statement of the American Diabetes Association (ADA) and the European Association for the Study of Diabetes (EASD). *Diabetes Care* 2012; 35:1364–1379

4. Inzucchi SE, Bergenstal RM, Buse JB, Diamant M, Ferrannini E, Nauck M, Peters AL, Tsapas A, Wender R, Matthews DR. Management of hyperglycemia in type 2 diabetes, 2015: a patient centered approach; update to a position statement of

the American Diabetes Association (ADA) and the European Association for the Study of Diabetes (EASD). *Diabetes Care* 2015;38:140–149

5. International Hypoglycaemia Study Group. Minimizing hypoglycemia in diabetes. *Diabetes Care* 2015;38:1583–1591

Index

Note: Page numbers followed by *f* refer to figures. Page numbers followed by *t* refer to tables. Page numbers in **bold** refer to an in-depth discussion.

F

G

I

J

K

L

M

N

O

T

U

V

W

Y